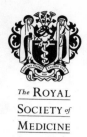

The ROYAL
SOCIETY *of*
MEDICINE

CW00621847

your guide to
asthma

Professor Stephen Holgate
MD, DSc, FRCP, FRCPath, FIBiol, FMed Sci

Professor Richard Beasley
MBChB, FRACP, DM, FAAAAI, FRCP

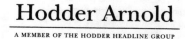

Hodder Arnold
A MEMBER OF THE HODDER HEADLINE GROUP

Orders: Please contact Bookpoint Ltd, 130 Milton Park,
Abingdon, Oxon OX14 4SB. Telephone: (44) 01235 827720,
Fax: (44) 01235 400454. Lines are open from 9.00 to
18.00, Monday to Saturday, with a 24-hour message
answering service. You can also order through our website
www.hoddereducation.com

British Library Cataloguing in Publication Data
A catalogue record for this title is available from the British
Library.

ISBN-10: 0 340 90619 7
ISBN-13: 9 780340 906194

First published   2005
Impression number   10 9 8 7 6 5 4 3 2 1
Year   2008 2007 2006 2005

Typeset by Servis Filmsetting Limited, Longsight, Manchester.
Printed in Great Britain for Hodder Arnold, a division of
Hodder Headline, 338 Euston Road, London NW1 3BH,
by Cox & Wyman Ltd, Reading, Berkshire.

Hodder Headline's policy is to use papers that are natural,
renewable and recyclable products and made from wood
grown in sustainable forests. The logging and manufacturing
processes are expected to conform to the environmental
regulations of the country of origin.

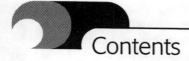

Contents

Acknowledgements

The authors would like to express their gratitude to Asthma UK for its support for this book. Asthma UK (formerly the National Asthma Campaign) is without doubt an outstanding organisation providing resources for people with asthma in the United Kingdom and internationally. It is an excellent source of independent professional advice and information to help people increase their understanding of asthma and reduce the effect of asthma on their lives. We have appreciated the opportunity of promoting the educational resources of Asthma UK in this book.

We would also like to thank Alison Pritchard and Denise Fabian of the Medical Research Institute of New Zealand, and Catherine Coe, Katie Archer and Lisa Collier of Hodder Arnold for their invaluable help in the successful completion of this project.

Stephen Holgate
Richard Beasley

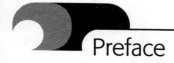
Preface

This new book, published in partnership with the Royal Society of Medicine, provides detailed, useful and up-to-date information on asthma. It contains expert yet user-friendly advice, with such useful features as:

Key Terms: demystifying the jargon
Questions and Answers: answering the burning questions
Myths and Facts: debunking the misconceptions
My Experience: how it feels to live with, or care for, someone with this condition.

Bearing the hallmark of excellence and accessibility that characterizes the work of the Royal Society of Medicine, this important guide will enable you and your family to gain some control over the way your asthma is managed by being better informed.

Peter Richardson
Director of Publications
Royal Society of Medicine

Introduction

Asthma is the most common of all lung diseases which affect all age groups. While most asthma starts in childhood, it can also occur at any time in life. It is a disorder in which the tubes that conduct air to and from the lungs become episodically narrowed, leading to wheeze, shortness of breath, cough and chest tightness. Most asthma is found in association with allergy to common environmental exposures such as house-dust mites, pets, pollen and fungi. These cause a special type of inflammation in the airways that makes them over-responsive to a wide range of stimuli that includes exercise, cold air, smoke and fumes. Asthmatic people are also more susceptible to attacks when they have the common cold. The consequences of asthma range from being an occasional nuisance to a severe disorder that greatly impacts on the quality of the affected person's daily life. Asthma that is inadequately controlled can be a frightening condition because the affected individual cannot easily anticipate when an attack will occur. This means that those affected often have a reduced recreational and social life as well as interference with school and work.

Affecting up to 10 per cent of adults and up to 20 per cent of children, asthma is not a trivial problem. Apart from its direct effects on people's lives, asthma is disruptive to families and costly both to the UK's National Health Service and personally. Unfortunately, asthma also carries a social stigma that compounds its influence on people's lives, especially those of children.

Asthma has not always been so common. From the 1960s there has been an enormous increase, especially in young people, that has been paralleled by a similar increase in other allergic disorders such as eczema, food allergy and hay fever. The cause for these rising trends is not known although recent research points to a strong link to the Western lifestyle. There is a greater proportion of children than adults with asthma, and it is clear that in many the disease improves through adolescent to early adult years. Asthma is often coinherited with allergy, but allergy alone is insufficient to cause the disease; it seems that an increased susceptibility of the lung itself to the environment is also needed.

For some people, asthma is only a temporary problem, particularly in a form more closely linked to a specific type of allergy that can be avoided. However, in others asthma may take on chronic and long-lasting characteristics. Apart from removal from a specific, known allergic trigger (for example, in the work place), there is no known cure for asthma. The disorder fluctuates in intensity, often being worse at specific times of the year in association with exposure to certain sensitizing allergens (for instance, pollens) or respiratory virus infections. Asthma may also get worse at times of stress, but it is important to note that it is not a psychological disorder. The fact that the disease cannot yet be cured does not mean that nothing can be done – indeed quite the opposite is true. Modern asthma management is highly effective. Most treatment is directed at reducing the inflammation in the airways so that they become less irritable. In addition to the regular use of these 'preventer' medications (usually inhaled steroids), rapid relief can be achieved with inhaled bronchodilators ('relievers').

The purpose of this book is to explain in a straightforward way the different types of asthma, their causes, diagnoses and treatment options. This information should give asthma sufferers and their families both the knowledge and confidence to manage their asthma effectively. We lay considerable emphasis on how those with asthma can self-manage their disease and, as a consequence, become less dependent upon medical help. Ultimately, this means that they will be able to cope with most aspects of their disease and learn to live with it rather than allow it to rule their lives. The primary object of treatment is to work towards returning lung function and daily activities to as normal a state as possible. Fortunately, there are now highly effective treatments, with new therapies coming along all the time.

There are many questions relating to asthma, and our overloaded health care system does not allow the necessary time for health professionals to answer all of these. We hope that this book will offer the kind of information and advice that people with asthma will find valuable, without too much medical jargon or scientific detail. We have tried to give clear answers to what are often difficult questions, where a simple 'yes' or 'no' answer is not known. This guide is written to provide the answers to the many questions people have asked us over the 30 or so years we have managed asthma patients. We hope that you find it interesting, informative and, above all, helpful.

CHAPTER

1

How many people have asthma?

The number of people with asthma

Asthma is a disease of modern life. It is common, with an estimated 300 million people affected worldwide. It has also become much more common since the 1960s. The number of people with asthma throughout the world has increased progressively since this time. This trend has been observed in both children and adults and in some countries the increase in the number of people with asthma has been dramatic. However, asthma is not the only allergic disorder that is becoming more common; associated allergic conditions such as eczema, hay fever and anaphylaxis are also becoming more common throughout the world. These trends are causing widespread concern, not least because we do not really understand the underlying reasons.

myth
Asthma is becoming more common due to worse air pollution

fact
It is not fully known why asthma rates are increasing and although air pollution contributes to the trends, it is not a major factor in asthma occurrence.

prevalence
The proportion of people with a condition in a defined population.

Q If I moved to a different part of the United Kingdom where asthma is not as much of a problem, would this improve my son's asthma, and help him to grow out of it?

A It is generally not recommended that families move in the hope that their children's asthma might improve, as there is no real evidence that this will help. Asthma varies from one person to another, so that a place that agrees with one person may not be so good for another. Except in a few circumstances, such as living in damp housing, there seems little to be gained by moving house.

The international patterns of asthma **prevalence** are shown on the world map (Figure 1.1). It shows that the United Kingdom has amongst the highest rates throughout the world, with asthma occurring in over one in ten children and one in twelve adults.

There are several other interesting observations that can also be made from the world asthma map. First, asthma appears to be more common in Western countries than in developing countries. However, asthma is now increasing at a fast rate in developing countries as they become more modernized and adopt Western lifestyles. Reassuringly it now appears that asthma rates have levelled off in many Western countries, such as the United Kingdom.

The map also shows that asthma varies significantly between different countries, even if they have the same predominant ethnic group and are close geographically. The best example of this is Hong Kong and Guangzhou in China, where Hong Kong has asthma rates that are four times higher than Guangzhou. This suggests that environmental or cultural factors have a large part to play in how common asthma is within different communities.

There is now an intensive research effort into the causes of asthma and over the next decade we are likely to gain a greater understanding of the causes of asthma, which will hopefully lead to preventive measures being taken which will reduce asthma rates.

Disability due to asthma

Asthma causes a considerable amount of disability throughout the world and much of it could be prevented with modern asthma

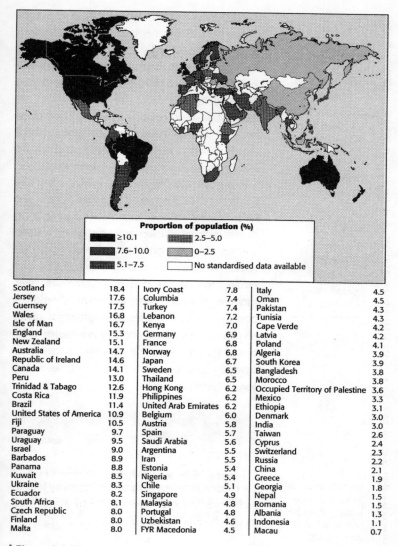

Proportion of population (%)

■ ≥10.1	▓ 2.5–5.0
▓ 7.6–10.0	░ 0–2.5
▓ 5.1–7.5	☐ No standardised data available

Scotland	18.4	Ivory Coast	7.8	Italy	4.5
Jersey	17.6	Columbia	7.4	Oman	4.5
Guernsey	17.5	Turkey	7.4	Pakistan	4.3
Wales	16.8	Lebanon	7.2	Tunisia	4.3
Isle of Man	16.7	Kenya	7.0	Cape Verde	4.2
England	15.3	Germany	6.9	Latvia	4.2
New Zealand	15.1	France	6.8	Poland	4.1
Australia	14.7	Norway	6.8	Algeria	3.9
Republic of Ireland	14.6	Japan	6.7	South Korea	3.9
Canada	14.1	Sweden	6.5	Bangladesh	3.8
Peru	13.0	Thailand	6.5	Morocco	3.8
Trinidad & Tabago	12.6	Hong Kong	6.2	Occupied Territory of Palestine	3.6
Costa Rica	11.9	Philippines	6.2	Mexico	3.3
Brazil	11.4	United Arab Emirates	6.2	Ethiopia	3.1
United States of America	10.9	Belgium	6.0	Denmark	3.0
Fiji	10.5	Austria	5.8	India	3.0
Paraguay	9.7	Spain	5.7	Taiwan	2.6
Uraguay	9.5	Saudi Arabia	5.6	Cyprus	2.4
Israel	9.0	Argentina	5.5	Switzerland	2.3
Barbados	8.9	Iran	5.5	Russia	2.2
Panama	8.8	Estonia	5.4	China	2.1
Kuwait	8.5	Nigeria	5.4	Greece	1.9
Ukraine	8.3	Chile	5.1	Georgia	1.8
Ecuador	8.2	Singapore	4.9	Nepal	1.5
South Africa	8.1	Malaysia	4.8	Romania	1.5
Czech Republic	8.0	Portugal	4.8	Albania	1.3
Finland	8.0	Uzbekistan	4.6	Indonesia	1.1
Malta	8.0	FYR Macedonia	4.5	Macau	0.7

Figure 1.1 World map of the prevalence of clinical asthma.

management. Even within Western Europe where the management of asthma is generally considered to be of a high standard, surveys have shown that around one in three people with asthma has disrupted sleep due to the illness at least once a week, and one in ten required an emergency hospital visit as a direct result of asthma in the previous year. In many regions of the world, asthma is one of the leading causes of hospital admissions in children.

In regions such as the Asia-Pacific, North and South America, Central and Eastern Europe and Africa, similar surveys have shown that disability due to asthma is even greater than in Western Europe. In these regions up to one in four people with asthma has severe attacks requiring hospital emergency care every year. However, with modern asthma management it should be possible to greatly reduce this high rate of severe attacks of asthma and improve the quality of life of asthmatics worldwide. There is a major gap between what can be achieved and the current level of asthma control.

myth
Asthma is generally well controlled.

fact
There is a huge gap between what can be achieved with modern asthma management and what is currently being achieved. Although effective treatment is available, people with asthma often do not benefit from it, leading to unnecessary suffering and even death. In the United Kingdom:

- ✧ Three out of four people with asthma experience symptoms needlessly
- ✧ Most deaths from asthma are 'preventable'
- ✧ One in six people with asthma reports weekly attacks so severe they cannot speak.

Death from asthma

At the beginning of the twentieth century it was widely considered that death from asthma was rare. A famous physician, William Osler, wrote in 1901 'The asthmatic pants into old age.' However, as asthma became more common during the second half of the twentieth century, deaths from asthma also became more common. It is estimated that asthma accounts for about one in 250 deaths worldwide. Currently in the United Kingdom around 1,400 people die from asthma every year.

> **myth**
> Asthma is merely a nuisance and not a serious illness.

> **fact**
> Asthma should be taken very seriously. In the United Kingdom:
>
> ◇ More than one in ten children and one in twelve adults suffer from asthma
> ◇ Around 70,000 hospital admissions every year are due to asthma
> ◇ Over 12 million working days are lost each year to asthma
> ◇ Around 1,400 people die from asthma each year.

The fact is that most deaths are preventable. In such cases there are often management problems that could easily have been overcome. This is why it is so important that asthma is managed correctly with the use of **preventive therapy**. Management problems fall into two groups: those relating to the day-to-day care and those relating to the treatment at the time of the life-threatening attack.

Problems associated with the day-to-day care are often caused by both the patient and doctor not realizing how severe their asthma is. Most

preventive therapy
Treatment that turns off the disease process in asthma, leading to improvements in asthma control with long-term use.

people with poorly controlled asthma do not recognize that they may be at risk of death. This problem is often made worse by patients seeing many different GPs (general practitioners) and not receiving regular medical care. As a result, inhaler medications are often used at the wrong times and incorrectly.

myth
Children don't die of asthma

fact
There is a widespread belief that children do not die from asthma. This view has come about because most communities have not experienced a child dying from asthma, despite asthma being very common. However, children do occasionally die from asthma, particularly teenagers and those from disadvantaged groups. One of the best ways to identify a child at risk of death is one who is taking lots of their bronchodilator inhaler (more than ten puffs per day, or requiring two or more inhalers per month), as this shows their asthma is out of control.

Similar problems have been found with the treatment of a severe attack that has subsequently led to death. In most cases, there is a lack of recognition by the patient, family or doctor of how severe the attack is. If someone does not recognize how serious an attack is, it results in a delay in seeking emergency medical services. Often in these situations, patients do not have an agreed management plan with instructions on when to seek medical care and what treatment to take. This results in them relying too much on their **bronchodilator (reliever) therapy** before seeking medical help. Chapters 5 and 6 look at overcoming these problems.

bronchodilator therapy
Medications that relax the airway muscle, leading to relief of airflow obstruction and symptoms of asthma over short periods. Bronchodilator therapy is often called 'reliever' therapy because it is used to relieve asthma symptoms.

Management problems that may lead to death

Long term

◇ Lack of appreciation of the severity of their asthma
◇ Not having or following a management plan
◇ Lack of regular medical care
◇ Preventive therapy used little or not at all.

Fatal attack

◇ Delay in seeking medical help
◇ Not recognizing the severity of the attack
◇ Over-reliance on bronchodilator (reliever) therapy
◇ Insufficient oral steroid use
◇ Lack of written guidelines for management.

The good news is that the death rate from asthma in the United Kingdom has progressively decreased over the last 15 years (Figure 1.2).

Q Why are people still dying from asthma?

A The main reason people die from asthma is because they do not recognize when they have developed a life-threatening asthma attack. Attacks can come on quickly or creep up slowly and the person may not be aware of the attack until it becomes very severe. Often patients gain a false sense of security from the temporary relief obtained from the repeated use of their inhaled 'reliever' bronchodilator. As a result patients tend to delay seeking medical help and do not receive adequate emergency treatment soon enough.

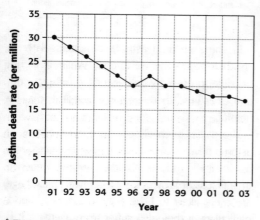

Figure 1.2 The reduction in the death rate from asthma in the United Kingdom since 1990.

Last year I had a close call when I ended up in the Intensive Care Unit with asthma. I had a bad attack but I thought I would be okay, as I had been previously. I struggled all night with my breathing but didn't call for help as I seemed to get relief from my bronchodilator inhaler. I must have gone through a whole inhaler over a 24-hour period, ending up taking it every five minutes or so. I finally called an ambulance which rushed me to hospital just in time. I have learnt my lesson and now have a written plan which tells me how to recognize when I get bad, and when to get medical care. The plan works really well and I now have a lot more confidence in dealing with a severe attack and won't put my life at risk again.

During this period, the death rate from asthma has fallen by almost half, a trend which is thought to be due to improvements in asthma management.

How does asthma develop?

Asthma usually first develops in childhood, although it can start at any age. There are several factors that influence the development of asthma. A viral chest infection called bronchiolitis (also known as croup) often leads to asthma. Exposure to tobacco smoke is also linked with wheezing in childhood. Babies who are breastfed are less likely to develop asthma or other allergies.

myth
Smoking during pregnancy does not increase the chance of the baby becoming asthmatic.

fact
Women who smoke during pregnancy are more likely to have babies who become asthmatic, as well as experiencing other serious lung illnesses such as pneumonia. They are also more likely to have a miscarriage, go into premature labour and give birth to babies who are lighter and have smaller lungs.

In some children asthma disappears later in childhood or early adulthood. While it is not possible to predict whether a child will grow out of their asthma, there are some clues that may be helpful.

The earlier in childhood that the symptoms of asthma develop, the more likely a child is to grow out of their asthma. Children who experience their first asthma symptoms after two years of age are more likely to have asthma into adulthood, particularly if they also suffer from allergies. It is thought that the presence of allergies is one of the reasons why asthma becomes persistent. Children with frequent severe attacks of asthma are less likely to grow out of their asthma than children with less severe disease.

Gender plays an important part in the development of asthma. Intriguingly, in infancy boys are more likely to develop asthma than girls; however, boys with asthma are more likely to grow out of their asthma than girls.

> **Q** **I have heard that some children can grow out of their asthma. Is this true?**
>
> **A** Yes. About half of all children with asthma will grow out of it by the time they become adults. This is more likely to occur if the child first develops asthma before they are two years old, never has really bad asthma attacks, is not allergic (does not have eczema or hay fever) and is a boy. However, in over a third of those who lose their asthma when young, symptoms return later in life.

> **Q** **Will my smoking affect my child's asthma?**
>
> **A** The simple answer to this question is yes. If you smoke, your child is more likely to get asthma and if your child already has asthma, it is likely to get worse. Asthma is not the only risk to your child, as exposure to tobacco smoke also reduces the growth of your baby's lungs and carries other risks such as cot death, pneumonia and more frequent ear infections.

An allergic child may have different allergic disorders at different stages of childhood, sometimes called the 'allergic march'. In infancy an allergy to food proteins such as milk and egg often leads to **eczema** (see Colour Plate 1). At around three years of age, the child may become allergic to allergens present in the air with the development of asthma. Later still, around the age of seven to ten years, the allergy to airborne allergens manifests as **rhinitis**, alongside asthma and this may also continue into adulthood. In such children it is likely that these illnesses represent different manifestations of the same underlying allergic tendency, being expressed in different parts of the body. Of course, all three conditions can co-exist in one child.

eczema
A skin condition that makes the skin dry and itchy.

rhinitis
An allergic condition of the nasal passages that causes a blocked and/or runny nose, and sneezing.

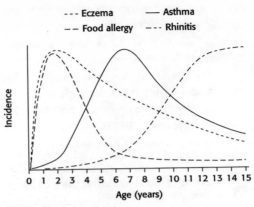

Figure 1.3 The allergic march.
Eczema usually presents in the first four years of life and is often (but not always) outgrown by the teenage years. Food allergy also begins before the age of two years, but is outgrown by the age of five years. Asthma develops later, usually between the ages of two and seven years. Allergic rhinitis presents later still, around the age of seven and, like asthma, may continue into adulthood.

For more information on the extent of asthma in the United Kingdom today, the document 'Where do we stand? Asthma in the UK today' will help:

www.asthma.org.uk/about/pdf/wheredowe stand.pdf

CHAPTER

2

What is asthma?

Definition

Asthma is a lung condition that has been recognized since ancient times, with references found in ancient Egyptian, Hebrew, Greek and Indian medical writings. The word *asthma* is derived from the Greek word αστμα meaning panting or short drawn breath. Asthma is defined as: 'A condition with widespread narrowing of the airways which changes in severity over short periods of time either spontaneously or with treatment.'

This definition describes the basic problem in asthma, which is the obstruction to the flow of air because of a narrowing of the **airways**. It also highlights the variability of asthma, in which patients get worse or better over short periods, depending on provoking or relieving factors.

airways
The tubes that carry air in and out of the lungs.

What causes the obstruction to airflow in asthma?

airway lumen
The space within the tubes through which air flows into and out of the lungs.

The obstruction to airflow that occurs in asthma is due to a number of processes which lead to a narrowing of the **lumen** of the airways.

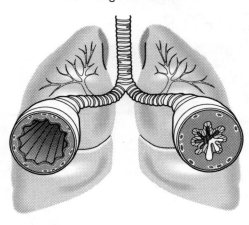

Figure 2.1 Airways in the normal state (left) and in asthma (right), demonstrating the narrowing of the airway lumen due to thickening of the airway wall and mucus, which leads to a greater resistance to the flow of air in and out of the lungs.

Bronchospasm

bronchospasm
The contraction of the airway (bronchial) muscles that leads to a narrowing of the airway lumen in asthma.

bronchial hyperresponsive-ness
The enhanced sensitivity of the airways in asthma, causing bronchospasm in response to irritants that do not normally affect people without asthma.

There are spirals of muscle that surround the major airways in the lungs. In someone who has asthma this muscle is thicker and more sensitive to triggers. A trigger will cause the muscle to tighten and, as it constricts, it makes the airways narrower. This is called **bronchospasm** and it may occur very quickly, for example in a person with asthma who walks out into cold air. Likewise, the muscle can be made to relax quickly by inhalation of a bronchodilator drug, which relieves the obstruction to airflow. In asthma the greater irritability of the airways is called **bronchial hyperresponsiveness**.

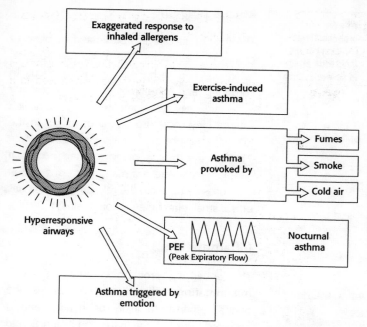

Figure 2.2 The hyperresponsive airways in asthma respond to a wide range of provoking factors.

Airway wall thickening

In asthma the airways are thicker than normal and, because they can only expand inwards rather than outwards, this leads to a narrowed lumen. The airway wall is thickened due to swelling caused by fluid from leaky blood vessels, the influx of inflammatory cells, thicker smooth muscle and a greater amount of connective scar tissue. Some components of this can be reversed by preventive drugs such as inhaled steroids.

inflammation
The process whereby the body responds to injury or irritation. It involves a complex series of events. Inflammation is the underlying problem in asthma. It is the main reason the airways in asthma are 'twitchy', responding to triggers that irritate them.

Mucus plugging

The flow of air can also be limited by plugs of mucus in the airways. The plugs may be thick, gelatinous and sticky, making them difficult to cough up, and sometimes completely blocking quite large airways. Sometimes a person with asthma may cough up a plug of mucus in the form of a cast of the airways (see Colour Plate 2). Extensive mucus plugging often occurs in people with severe asthma, and means that at the doses being taken the reliever medicine has only a small effect (see Colour Plate 3).

Inflammation

The underlying problem causing asthma is **inflammation**. Inflammation represents the body's response to injury or irritation and is designed to restore the tissue and its function to normal and then switch itself off. However, in some conditions such as asthma, this inflammatory process may damage the tissue, badly affect its function and not switch off, which causes persistent problems.

Another common disease in which this occurs is rheumatoid arthritis in which inflammation causes redness and swelling of the joints, which persists and gets worse over time, causing damage to the joints and resulting in stiffness and deformity. In asthma the swelling and redness resulting from inflammation in the airways can be seen by looking directly into the lungs, as shown in Colour Plate 4.

fact
Even when a person with asthma feels well and has few symptoms, they still have an active inflammatory process in their airways. This is one of the reasons why people with asthma are encouraged to take their preventive therapy regularly all the time, not just when their asthma is unstable.

Q Would it be advisable not to own a cat or a dog to reduce the risk of my children having allergies such as asthma?

A Children are at no greater risk of developing asthma if there is a cat or dog in the household. However, if your child already has asthma and is allergic to cats or dogs, then exposure may provoke their asthma symptoms. As a result it is wise not to get a cat or dog if your child already has asthma.

Risk factors for asthma

There are numerous risk factors that have been shown to increase the chances of developing asthma. Some of these are influenced by lifestyle, but it is clear that many of the factors cannot be influenced at all. Other factors, such as breastfeeding, can reduce the risk of a child developing asthma. The factors that influence the risk of developing asthma include:

✧ A family history of asthma
✧ **Allergen** exposure – indoor and outdoor
✧ Smoking – active and passive
✧ Small family size
✧ Air pollution – indoor and outdoor
✧ Diet
✧ Drugs
✧ Obesity
✧ Occupational exposures.

allergen
A substance that may provoke an allergic response in a susceptible person. Common allergens include house-dust mites, grass pollen and cat dander.

fact
Asthma is a physical condition and is no more common in people with psychiatric or psychological conditions. However, emotional stress can trigger symptoms in sufferers, and psychological problems can lead to difficulties in the management of asthma.

house-dust mite
Tiny creatures invisible to the naked eye that live in the dust that builds up around the house, in particular in mattresses, carpets and soft furnishings. Most people with asthma are allergic to the faeces from the house-dust mite.

pollen
The tiny grains given off by grasses, flowers and trees. Most people with rhinitis, and many with asthma, are allergic to pollens.

immunoglobulin E (IgE)
The antibody which is involved in allergic responses.

Q What climate or environment is best for a person with asthma?

A This is very specific to each individual. No one climate or environment is ideal for all people with asthma, since there are so many triggers relating to different climatic factors. If you move to another area, climatic factors relating to the new environment may still provoke your asthma symptoms.

Classification of asthma

Over the years the classification of asthma has changed as the understanding of asthma has increased:

Extrinsic v. intrinsic asthma

The original classification of asthma was that there were two forms:

Extrinsic asthma – this is asthma caused by exposure to external factors such as inhaled allergens.

Intrinsic asthma – this is due to internal factors such as infections or psychological factors.

Atopic v. non-atopic asthma

Following the extrinsic or intrinsic classification of asthma, the ability to measure sensitivity to allergens such as **house-dust mites** or **pollens** by allergy skin prick tests or blood **IgE** tests was developed. This led to the subsequent classification of atopic or non-atopic asthma, depending on whether the allergy tests were positive or negative.

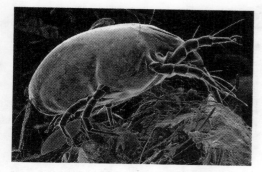

Figure 2.3 A house-dust mite magnified 500 times.

The atopic versus non-atopic classification of asthma led to the study of the role of allergens in the development of asthma to find out whether avoiding allergens could lead to better controlled asthma. Despite early promise, such allergen avoidance studies have generally been disappointing in terms of leading to marked improvements in asthma control.

Severity

More recently asthma has been classified according to its severity. The reasoning behind this approach is that treatment is based on asthma severity and that if the patient is classified correctly they are more likely to receive the right treatment. In this way, people with asthma are considered to have either persistent or intermittent asthma, depending on whether their **symptoms** occur on most days (persistent) or only occasionally (intermittent). Persistent asthma sufferers are further classified into mild, moderate and severe, depending on the level of their symptoms, lung function impairment and the amount of treatment required to control their asthma.

symptom
A sensation experienced by an individual as a result of an illness or problem. The symptoms of asthma include breathlessness, wheezing, coughing and chest tightness.

Table 1 Classification of asthma severity by clinical features before starting treatment

1	**Intermittent**	• Occasional brief symptoms (<1–2 times/week during day; <1–2 times/month at night) • Peak flow >80% predicted and variability <20%.
2	**Mild persistent**	• Symptoms (<1 time/day but >1–2 times/week during the day; <1 time/week but >1–2 times/month at night) • Peak flow >70–80% predicted and variability <20–30%.
3	**Moderate persistent**	• Daily symptoms, symptoms at night >1 time/week • Peak flow >60–70% predicted and variability >30%.
4	**Severe persistent**	• Daily symptoms • Frequent symptoms at night • Limitation of daily activities • Peak flow <60% predicted and variability >30%.

Patients in all severity grades can experience severe attacks of asthma. However, the frequency and severity of attacks is likely to be greater for those whose asthma is classed as severe to begin with.

Factors that provoke asthma

One of the features of asthma is that the airways are too sensitive to a wide range of stimuli, as outlined in the bulleted list below. The stimuli do not cause asthma in the first place, but bring on the symptoms or attacks of asthma in a person with asthma. This irritable state of the airways is referred to as hyperresponsiveness.

my experience

Having had asthma for 25 years I know most of the things that make it worse. Dust, perfume and smoke always make me wheeze and so I try to avoid situations with these exposures. I get asthma when I exercise and so I take a puff of my reliever inhaler before I go jogging. I know that a cold is likely to provoke a bad attack, so I go along to see my doctor when symptoms of a cold first occur.

Stimuli that can provoke asthma symptoms

✧ Cold air
✧ Exercise
✧ Climate, including changes in temperature and humidity, e.g. fog
✧ Air pollution, both indoor and outdoor
✧ Fumes, including smoke, perfume, sprays
✧ Allergens, including house-dust mite, cat, dog, moulds
✧ Medications, including
  – beta blockers used for heart disease and high blood pressure
  – non-steroidal anti-inflammatory drugs such as aspirin used for pain relief or arthritis
✧ Emotion, including stress and loss (bereavement)
✧ Hormonal, such as premenstrual and during pregnancy
✧ Night time and early morning
✧ Foods, including preservatives, such as tartrazine (orange colouring), MSG (used in Chinese food), sulphites (included in some wines) and allergens such as peanuts and shellfish
✧ Workplace exposure to agents to which individuals become sensitized
✧ Alcohol
✧ Viral respiratory tract infections such as the common cold and influenza.

These provoking factors signal to the patient the presence of various problems, for example, if asthma symptoms are frequently triggered by exercise, fumes or night time (**nocturnal asthma**), this is a sign of unstable asthma.

Q Why is asthma often worse at night?

A As part of the normal 'body clock' everyone has a reduction in lung function at night — the problem in asthma sufferers is that this fall is greater and can lead to difficulties. Changes in air and body temperature, increased acid production by the stomach, low levels of body hormones at night, the loss of the effect of asthma drugs taken earlier in the day and even greater exposure to house-dust mite in the bedding can all make asthma worse. If a sufferer's symptoms are worse at night or first thing in the morning, it is a sign that their asthma is unstable and that they probably require an increase in their regular preventive therapy.

nocturnal asthma
Asthma symptoms which occur at night. It is a sign that asthma is not under adequate control, even if asthma symptoms are not a problem during the day.

Changes in climate can trigger asthma symptoms through changes in temperature and humidity as well as other factors such as the release of allergenic pollen particles, especially after thunder storms. The focus on air pollution is often on outdoor sources such as vehicle exhaust fumes, however, indoor sources from cooking or heating with natural gas, coal or wood are also important, as are household varnishes, solvents and cleaning chemicals, particularly in those who spend most of their time indoors.

Similarly, both indoor and outdoor allergens can provoke asthma symptoms. The most common allergens that people with asthma are sensitized to are house-dust mites, cat and dog dander, cockroaches, pollens and moulds, as shown in Figure 2.4. While it is not possible to completely avoid these allergens, a person is able to reduce the level of exposure, which is covered in Chapter 5.

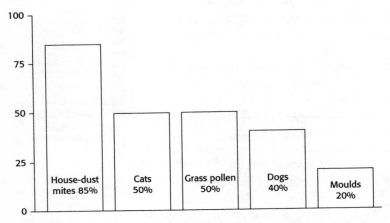

Figure 2.4 Proportions of asthmatic children sensitized to the common allergens.

Asthma can also be provoked by a wide range of foods, additives and preservatives which usually can only be identified by careful monitoring. These include foods to which a person may be allergic, such as egg, peanuts and shellfish, preservatives such as tartrazine (orange colouring) and sulphites (in certain alcoholic drinks such as wine) and foods such as some fruits. In some young children asthma may be affected by other foods such as milk and wheat, in which case eczema may also occur. Working out if a specific food provokes asthma is difficult, requiring careful monitoring by the patient. Interestingly a recent international study has reported that people in countries with a high intake of fresh fruit and vegetables may be protected from developing asthma. Together with the general health benefits of such a diet, it can also be recommended for children who may be at risk of developing asthma.

myth
Diet does not affect asthma.

fact
There is a general view that it is only irritants that can be breathed in that can provoke asthma and that diet is not important. This is not true, however, for although in most people with asthma its severity is not related to their diet, there is a number of situations where specific foods can make asthma worse.

Patterns of attacks

Severe **attacks** of asthma can happen in different ways. Three main patterns have been recognized.

asthma attack
An episode of severe asthma in which a person has difficulty breathing. The cause of the attack and its presentation may vary.

1 A sudden attack in which the asthmatic patient develops severe asthma within minutes or hours of the onset of the first symptoms. This type is called a precipitate attack.
2 A severe attack which occurs quickly after a few days of unstable asthma.
3 An attack in which there is a gradual worsening evolving over several days to weeks, leading progressively to more severe asthma.

fact

Most attacks of asthma develop after a period of worsening control that has occurred over a day or more. The reason people with asthma often think that the attack has come on suddenly is that they do not recognize that their asthma has become progressively worse. This is partly because the sensations from the chest may not be recognized and people with worsening asthma learn to restrict their activities when their asthma worsens, which limits the impact of the problem.

The most common causes of severe attacks of asthma are viral respiratory tract infections (such as a cold or the flu), heavy allergen exposure (outdoor or indoor) or if certain medications are taken (such as aspirin or other anti-inflammatory drugs). Another important cause of worsening asthma with more frequent attacks is patients not taking their preventive (controller) treatment (usually inhaled steroids) regularly or even stopping their treatment. It is always worthwhile trying to work out what causes a severe attack, so that it can be avoided whenever possible in the future.

The high-risk asthmatic

Any person who suffers from asthma can have a severe attack which may threaten their life. However, some people with asthma are at considerably greater risk than others and can be identified if they have one or more risk factors from the following list:

- ✧ Adolescents
- ✧ Disadvantaged racial groups
- ✧ Those with psychological or psychosocial problems
- ✧ Those who have three or more asthma medications prescribed
- ✧ Those who require more than two reliever bronchodilator inhalers per month
- ✧ People who make frequent visits to their GP for unstable asthma
- ✧ People who have needed one or more hospital emergency department visits in the last year

✧ Anyone with a recent hospital admission for asthma

✧ Sufferer who has had a previous admission to an Intensive Care Unit (ICU) or High Dependency Unit (HDU) for asthma.

> **my experience**
>
> I usually ring my GP for repeat prescriptions of my bronchodilator inhaler when I run out and I go along and pick them up without having to see her. However, at one time when I was using a lot of my bronchodilator inhaler and asked for a second repeat in a month she asked me to go and see her, as she thought I was 'at risk'. She persuaded me to go back on my preventive inhaler rather than relying on my bronchodilator one, and now my asthma is a lot better and I hardly need to use my bronchodilator inhaler at all.

The markers of risk relate either to factors that negatively affect behaviour or access to medical care, or to underlying past asthma severity. The greater the number of risk factors present, the greater the risk of a life-threatening attack. 'High-risk' patients should see their doctor regularly.

CHAPTER

3

How is asthma diagnosed?

Diagnosis

A doctor normally makes a diagnosis of asthma from the patient's description of their symptoms, together with a short physical examination. The diagnosis is then confirmed by breathing tests which show the characteristic variable pattern of lung function. There is no blood test or x-ray that can confirm the diagnosis of asthma.

Asthma symptoms

The characteristic symptoms described by people with asthma are:

✧ **Wheezing**
✧ Tightness in the chest
✧ Coughing
✧ Breathlessness.

These symptoms are triggered by different factors which irritate the sensitive airways, particularly:

◇ Night or early morning
◇ Exercise or cold air
◇ **Viral respiratory tract infection**
◇ Exposure to allergens, e.g. house-dust mite, cat fur
◇ Exposure to non-specific irritants, e.g. cigarette smoke, perfumes
◇ Drugs, e.g. beta blockers, aspirin
◇ Emotion or stress
◇ Occupational exposure.

Q How can I tell if my child has asthma?

A A child with asthma is likely to have recurrent wheezing, coughing and breathlessness which comes and goes in different circumstances. Usually the symptoms are more noticeable at night or early morning, in the cold or after exercise, with more severe episodes occurring when your child is suffering from a cold.

There is a number of points that the doctor will need to consider before diagnosing a patient with asthma. Not all the symptoms may be present in one person, or some symptoms may be more dominant. The occurrence of wheezing is the most important symptom to enable the diagnosis of asthma to be made. The doctor will also take into account that some of the symptoms of asthma can occur in a wide range of other respiratory conditions as given on page 29.

wheeze
A whistling sound made by a person who has airflow obstruction when breathing. In a person with asthma wheezing is high-pitched, and is usually heard when breathing out, although if airflow obstruction is severe it may also occur when breathing in. If a person with very severe asthma stops wheezing, this is a serious sign as it means the airways have narrowed so much that there is not enough air passing through them to make the wheezing sound.

viral respiratory tract infection
An infection of the respiratory tract caused by a virus. The site and severity of the illness may vary depending on the specific virus, ranging from a runny nose due to the common cold, to an illness with fever, aching, breathlessness and coughing due to the influenza virus.

myth
Wheezing always indicates asthma.

fact
Wheezing normally indicates asthma, particularly if it is recurrent. However, there are other short-term conditions (such as infective bronchitis) and long-term conditions (such as chronic bronchitis and emphysema in the elderly) which may also cause wheezing.

The presence and frequency of some symptoms such as waking at night may help in determining the severity of asthma.

Examination

Clinical examination of the patient is helpful in confirming the diagnosis of asthma if wheezing is present at the time of the consultation. Wheezing is the main sign of asthma and to recognize it the doctor will listen carefully for the whistling sound through a stethoscope placed on the patient's chest as the patient breathes in and out. As airflow obstruction in asthma is not there all the time, wheezing may not necessarily be present during the consultation.

The physical examination also provides the opportunity for the doctor to look for signs of other allergic conditions such as eczema, and evidence of other disorders that may be similar to asthma.

Lung function tests

Lung function tests will demonstrate whether there is **reversible airflow obstruction**. Several approaches may be used, depending on the situation.

1 Home peak flow monitoring

This involves repeat measurements of the **peak flow** at different times of the day and night, before and after a bronchodilator. The peak flow is measured on a peak flow meter (see Chapter 4). If the highest and lowest peak flows vary by more than 15 per cent this indicates that variable airflow

reversible airflow obstruction
Airflow obstruction that comes and goes over short periods, being worse with provoking stimuli (such as cold air) and resolving with treatment (such as inhaled bronchodilator).

peak flow
The maximum speed at which air can be forced out of the lungs. It is a sensitive measure of the severity of the obstruction to the flow of air in a person with asthma.

obstruction is present and that it is likely that the person has asthma.

This period of monitoring is useful not only in confirming the diagnosis of asthma, but also in looking at how the changes in peak flow relate to the symptoms experienced by the person with asthma. Normally a diary card is used for the patient to enter their peak flow readings and symptoms. It is usually easy for both the doctor and the patient to tell from the diary how severe the patient's asthma is. A peak flow chart may also help to establish the underlying cause of asthma with worsening in special circumstances, for example, asthma caused by exposure to chemicals or allergens in the workplace.

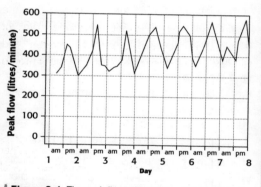

Figure 3.1 The peak flow record of an untreated patient with asthma shows characteristic variability, being worse in the early morning and better in the late afternoon.

myth
Peak flow meters are expensive and difficult to use.

fact
In many countries, including the United Kingdom, peak flow meters are funded by the government. As a result, they should be available free of charge from your doctor or nurse. Peak flow meters are very simple to use.

Q What is the best test that a patient can have to confirm the diagnosis of asthma?

A The best way to confirm the diagnosis is for the patient to repeatedly measure their lung function using a peak flow meter. If the peak flow measurements are low first thing in the morning, in the cold or after exercise, and are higher at other times of the day then it is likely that the patient has asthma. Another way to confirm the diagnosis of asthma is to see if the peak flow increases after taking a few puffs of a bronchodilator inhaler.

2 Bronchodilator responsiveness

An alternative method which may be used in the doctor's surgery is to measure the improvement in lung function in response to a bronchodilator reliever medication. This involves measuring the lung function both before and after using a bronchodilator. The diagnosis of asthma is then confirmed in individuals in whom the peak flow improves by more than 15 per cent of the starting value. The lack of such an improvement does not necessarily mean that the patient does not have asthma; instead he or she may not have airflow obstruction at the time of the test, may have already taken a bronchodilator before the test, or may have partially reversible airflow obstruction. It is then necessary to confirm the diagnosis using home peak flow monitoring.

Assessment of bronchodilator responsiveness is most helpful if the peak flow is low to start with, although it is worth doing in all individuals at the time the diagnosis is considered as it will enable the doctor to determine the maximum peak flow rate.

3 Response to inhaled steroid treatment

This approach can be used with some patients who appear to have irreversible airflow obstruction and in which the diagnosis has not been confirmed by either of the above methods. It involves the measurement of lung function such as peak flow before and after a one to two month trial of inhaled steroids. This is the most effective preventive medication available to achieve long-term asthma control and therefore if there is no change with its use, it is most likely that the person does not have asthma.

4 Response to exercise

Another approach is to determine the change in peak flow in response to exercise which is the most common trigger that can provoke asthma. This method is primarily used in children who are well at the time and, as a result, it may be difficult to confirm the diagnosis of asthma. The child's peak flow is recorded and then the child runs for six minutes with a peak flow being recorded every ten minutes for thirty minutes after stopping. A fall in peak flow of more than 15 per cent would confirm the diagnosis of asthma. This is referred to as exercise-induced asthma, and is discussed in more detail in Chapter 7.

Other diagnoses

In older adults there is another common condition called **chronic obstructive pulmonary disease** (also known as COPD) which has similar symptoms to asthma. COPD covers two conditions: **chronic (persistent) bronchitis** and **emphysema**. COPD usually results from long-term exposure to irritants to the lungs, such as cigarette smoking, workplace irritants and air pollution. Tobacco smoking is by far the most important cause.

The feature which differentiates COPD from asthma is that in asthma the airflow obstruction (and as a result the symptoms and lung function) varies, whereas in COPD the airflow obstruction is usually irreversible, with little change in either symptoms or lung function between days. Chronic bronchitis patients have a persistent cough which produces phlegm every day; in those with emphysema, breathlessness is the dominant symptom.

chronic obstructive pulmonary disease (COPD)
A group of slowly progressive respiratory conditions resulting from long-term exposure to irritants to the lung such as smoking. COPD is characterized by airflow obstruction that does not fully reverse and is associated with infective episodes, especially in the winter months.

chronic bronchitis
A disease which is characterized by the over-production of phlegm in response to long-term exposure to irritants (such as smoking). People with chronic bronchitis have a persistent cough with phlegm, as well as wheezing.

emphysema
A disease in which the lung is progressively destroyed due to exposure to irritants (such as smoking). It is characterized by breathlessness which limits daily activities.

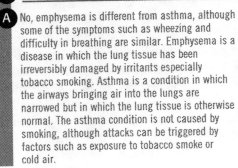

Q Is emphysema the same as asthma?

A No, emphysema is different from asthma, although some of the symptoms such as wheezing and difficulty in breathing are similar. Emphysema is a disease in which the lung tissue has been irreversibly damaged by irritants especially tobacco smoking. Asthma is a condition in which the airways bringing air into the lungs are narrowed but in which the lung tissue is otherwise normal. The asthma condition is not caused by smoking, although attacks can be triggered by factors such as exposure to tobacco smoke or cold air.

Many patients with COPD have features of both chronic bronchitis and emphysema as well as an 'asthmatic component' which means that they respond to some degree to bronchodilator therapy. Due to the overlap of these three conditions people with COPD are often given a trial of asthma medications.

Q Why have I been given asthma inhalers if I have emphysema and chronic bronchitis, but not asthma?

A The reliever bronchodilator inhalers used in asthma may also provide some benefit to patients with emphysema and chronic bronchitis. Although the benefit is not as great in emphysema and in chronic bronchitis as it is in asthma, these medications are still worthy of a trial. The reliever bronchodilator inhalers may provide some welcome relief from the breathlessness experienced, even if there is little improvement in lung function.

There is a wide range of other illnesses affecting the lungs which share some of the symptoms of asthma, in particular intermittent breathlessness and cough. In addition to COPD these include infections such as tuberculosis and bronchiectasis (in which the phlegm is discoloured and patients may have a fever, which is uncommon in asthma), lung cancer (which may also lead to weight loss and coughing up blood, which again does not normally occur in asthma) and heart failure (in which congestion in the lungs may cause similar symptoms). In a situation where doctors suspect another condition it is likely that the patient will undergo a chest x-ray.

CHAPTER

4

What tests are helpful?

Lung function

There are a number of different reasons for measuring lung function in a person with asthma. A doctor may use this approach to help confirm the diagnosis of asthma and to give an estimate of the severity at the time of measurement. When measured by patients themselves, it gives them the ability to monitor the control of their asthma.

Devices

When people with asthma measure their lung function at home they usually use a device called a peak flow meter. This is a simple device which measures the peak flow (see Chapter 3); when the airways narrow, the peak flow falls.

The best way to use a **peak flow meter** is to:

1 Sit upright.
2 Slide marker hard up to the beginning of the groove.
3 Hold meter level.
4 Keep fingers clear of marker.
5 Take a deep breath in.
6 Close your lips around the mouthpiece.
7 Huff out hard and fast.
8 Read where the marker is on the scale.
9 Repeat these steps three times.
10 Record the best of the three readings.

> **peak flow meter**
> A device which measures the maximum speed at which air can be forced out of the lungs.

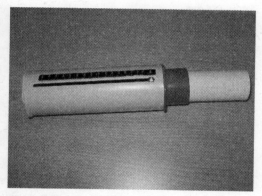

Figure 4.1 A peak flow meter.

The other commonly used device is a spirometer which measures the **FEV$_1$**. With airway narrowing in asthma it is more difficult to blow out as quickly as normal, and as a result the FEV$_1$ is reduced.

> **FEV$_1$**
> The forced expiratory volume in one second — the amount of air that can be forced out of the lungs in one second.

The peak flow meter and spirometer are easy to use and, because most practitioners are familiar with the techniques involved, they are the lung function measurements most commonly used in clinical practice. However, due to the large size and cost of the equipment, spirometry is normally reserved for use in hospitals or in doctors' surgeries.

fact
The predicted peak flow values will depend on the person's age, gender and height. As a result, to find out a person's 'predicted' peak flow it is necessary to refer to standard reference tables (see Figure 4.3).

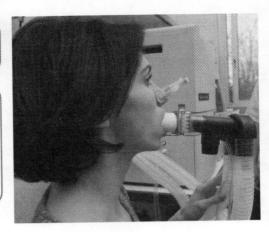

Figure 4.2 A spirometer.

Diagnosis

The purpose of using lung function tests to make the diagnosis of asthma is to identify if there is significant variation either with repeat measurements at home or in response to bronchodilator treatment (see Chapter 3).

Monitoring control

Lung function measurements can be really helpful in enabling patients with asthma to know how well controlled their asthma is. This approach can help overcome the difficulty many patients have in trying to tell how bad their asthma is by how they feel. In one study it was shown that about one in four adult patients with asthma may have minimal or no breathlessness, despite lung function values falling to less than 50 per cent of normal. Alarmingly, it is often the most severe asthmatic patients who have the worst perception of the severity of their asthma, i.e. those at greatest risk are least likely to recognize a severe attack.

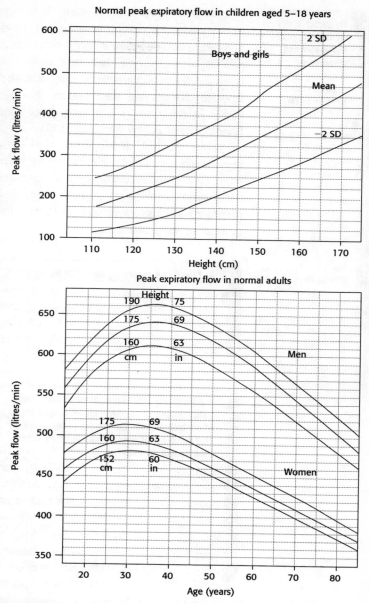

Figure 4.3 Standard tables for peak flow in children (top) and adults (bottom). A total of 95 per cent of all children will have a peak flow value between the 2SD and −2SD lines.

Q My doctor wants me to get a peak flow meter and measure my breathing capacity at home – do I need to do this?

A Yes. Many people with asthma have difficulty recognizing how bad their asthma is by how they feel. This may be a problem as asthma can get worse quickly and if a patient with asthma cannot tell how severe it is they may delay in seeking medical treatment. This can be helped by keeping an eye on your peak flow rates and following a written plan, whereby you know what to do when your peak flow falls.

To help overcome this problem it is now recommended that patients have the opportunity to measure their peak flow at home. This enables patients to know how well their asthma is controlled. It also allows patients to know at what stage to change their treatment, or see their doctor in the case of a severe attack (see Appendix for peak flow diary, page 112).

Asthma UK has developed a peak flow diary which can be downloaded from www.asthma.org.uk/about/control.php. It also provides background information about peak flow monitoring and instructions on what to do in the event of an attack of asthma.

Q Do I need to measure my peak flow all the time?

A For most people with asthma it is usually not necessary to measure the peak flow every day. After an initial period of monitoring, it is better to focus on measuring your peak flow at times when your asthma is unstable.

Q Are there any other medical conditions where patients have to regularly measure their level of control, and use the results to help work out how much medication to take or when to see their doctor urgently?

A The best example is diabetes. It is often difficult for patients with diabetes to know how low or high their blood sugar levels are and, as a result, how well controlled their diabetes is and how much insulin they need to take. It is for this reason that diabetics are encouraged to measure their blood sugar levels regularly and to change their insulin dose depending on their blood sugar level, according to a pre-determined plan.

Other investigations

Alternative diagnoses

The tests that might be used to exclude or confirm alternative diagnoses will depend on what conditions are suspected. The test which is most likely to be ordered in this situation is a chest x-ray. The chest x-ray almost always appears normal in uncomplicated asthma, and so a doctor is only likely to order this if another condition is suspected. If the chest x-ray is abnormal a more detailed x-ray, called a CT (computerized tomography) scan, may then be undertaken to define the problem more clearly.

More detailed breathing tests may be undertaken to investigate other causes of abnormal lung function. The equipment required for these detailed lung function tests is considerably more expensive and difficult to use than the peak flow meter or spirometer, and as a result, these tests are normally undertaken in a hospital-based specialist clinic.

One of the detailed lung function tests which may be required to confirm or rule out the diagnosis of asthma is the bronchial challenge test. In this test patients inhale increasingly higher concentrations of an irritant substance such as histamine or methacholine. Depending on the dose required to provoke asthma, the probability of the person having asthma can be determined. Due to the risks and difficulty in performing and interpreting bronchial challenge tests, it is not routinely used in the diagnosis of asthma. However, it is helpful in specific situations such as the assessment of the risk of diving for a person with asthma, when person has unusual

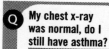

Q My chest x-ray was normal, do I still have asthma?

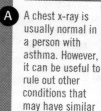

A A chest x-ray is usually normal in a person with asthma. However, it can be useful to rule out other conditions that may have similar symptoms to asthma.

symptoms of asthma, for example, chronic cough, and the confirmation of an asthmatic reaction to a workplace agent suspected of causing asthma.

A **sputum** sample is normally taken if a chest infection is suspected to find out what type it is and what antibiotic to use. Alternatively, a sputum sample might be taken if, for example, lung cancer was suspected, in which case it would be examined for cancer cells.

Blood tests may be required in certain circumstances. For example, a full blood count may be undertaken to measure the level of the allergic white cells (eosinophils), which play an important role in the airways inflammation in asthma. People with asthma taking a medication called theophylline require occasional blood tests to check the level of this medication.

Allergen sensitivity

Skin prick testing and the measurement of serum IgE represent the two main methods to detect the specific allergens to which a person with asthma may be sensitized. Skin prick testing is the preferred method as it is simple, safe and relatively cheap to perform, and the results are available immediately (see Colour Plate 5). Identifying the allergens to which a person with asthma is sensitized enables avoidance measures to be put into place to reduce exposure.

Measuring the presence of IgE antibodies to specific allergens is an alternative to skin prick testing but is more costly and requires a blood test that needs to be sent to a special laboratory

---

sputum

The thick mucus which is coughed up by a person. It is also commonly called phlegm.

---

skin prick test

A test to find out whether a person is sensitive to specific allergens. Drops of allergen are placed on the skin, the skin is then pricked through the allergen solution, and the size of the resulting skin swelling is measured.

which delays the results. It is normally reserved for patients who have bad eczema, those who cannot be withdrawn from medications which interfere with skin prick testing, for example antihistamines, or when the patient is at risk of a major adverse reaction from skin prick testing.

my experience

I always thought that I was an 'allergic' person but it was only after I had skin prick tests that I knew what I was definitely allergic to. The skin prick tests have been really helpful in allowing me to know which allergens to try to avoid.

myth

A positive allergen skin prick test means that the allergen is the underlying cause of your asthma.

fact

A positive allergen skin prick test indicates that exposure to that particular allergen may provoke asthma, but not that it is necessarily the underlying cause of asthma. People without asthma can also have positive skin prick tests. Indeed, about 30 per cent of people in developed countries have positive skin prick tests, whereas between 5 and 15 per cent have asthma.

Associated conditions

There are several investigations which may be required depending on the clinical situation. One condition which is commonly associated with asthma is reflux oesophagitis, which is the cause of heartburn. In reflux oesophagitis, acid from the stomach flows back into the oesophagus and may also irritate the airways and contribute to unstable asthma. This association is important to recognize in a person with asthma, for if they receive treatment for reflux oesophagitis it may help their asthma to improve.

Chronic sinusitis is another condition commonly associated with asthma (see Chapter 7). A standard test to define the nature and extent of sinusitis is a CT scan (see Colour Plate 6).

An uncommon disorder that occurs in people with severe asthma is allergic bronchopulmonary aspergillosis (ABPA for short). ABPA, which develops as a result of an unusual type of allergy to a mould called *Aspergillus* is difficult to diagnose and requires a series of blood tests, skin prick tests, sputum examination, as well as a CT scan. These tests are normally undertaken in a person with severe asthma who appears to be getting frequent chest infections and is not responding to treatment.

Potential complications

A range of tests may be required in the more severe asthmatic patient to investigate the potential complications of asthma or its treatment. The most common test undertaken is measurement of bone mineral density in patients who require frequent, or continuous, courses of oral steroid therapy as they may have developed thin bones (**osteoporosis**). Specialized x-ray techniques can measure the density of bone at different sites in the body, such as the spine and hip. With the availability of a new class of oral medications called bisphosphonates, it is now possible to treat people who have developed thin bones.

Another test which is carried out on people with asthma who have required high doses of oral steroids is the synacthen test. This test measures the function of the adrenal gland, which makes a hormone called cortisol which is essential for normal health. Levels of cortisol may be reduced with prolonged oral steroid treatment, leading to tiredness, aching and nausea. The synacthen test involves an injection with a hormone that stimulates the adrenal gland, with the resulting cortisol response measured with blood tests.

osteoporosis
A condition characterized by thin bones which can result in fractures. Osteoporosis can be caused by long-term oral steroid therapy and is treated by a class of medications called bisphosphonates.

my experience

I have had severe asthma for most of my life, with too many hospital admissions to count. I eventually went on continuous oral steroids, taking prednisolone 7.5 mg every day. I didn't like this, but realized it was necessary to keep me alive. My doctor gets my bone density measured every three years, but I don't seem to have a problem with thin bones. However, my adrenal glands are suppressed and I know that I can get sick if I ever miss my daily dose. I also know I need to double the dose of prednisolone to 15 mg every day if I'm sick for any reason such as if I get the flu. I also wear a Medic Alert bracelet indicating that I'm on long-term oral steroids and have adrenal suppression.

CHAPTER

5

Treatment

Aims

The aims of the long-term management of asthma are to:

⟡ Control symptoms including night time symptoms and exercise-induced asthma
⟡ Achieve the best possible lung function
⟡ Prevent severe attacks, in particular life-threatening attacks that lead to hospital admission
⟡ Ensure there are minimal side effects from the medications used.

It is not possible to specify the exact level of lung function or symptom control that should be achieved, as this will depend on how severe a patient's asthma is. It also depends on the goals and preferences of both the patient and the doctor. Notwithstanding this caution, most people with asthma can control it well with modern asthma management.

Medications

There are two major types of medications used in the treatment of asthma: **bronchodilator drugs** and **preventive drugs**. Generally, the number, dose and frequency of use of both types of medications increase as asthma becomes more severe. Most anti-asthma drugs are taken by inhalation because this improves their effectiveness and at the same time reduces side effects. In the case of bronchodilators, the inhaled route also increases the speed of onset of the effect.

Bronchodilator drugs

Bronchodilator drugs act by relaxing the muscles around the airways, which helps the airways to open up, so making it easier to breathe. There are several types of bronchodilators of which short-acting beta agonist drugs are the most commonly used.

Short-acting beta agonist drugs

Short-acting beta agonist drugs are bronchodilators normally taken through an **inhaler** device, start working within a few minutes and last for about four to six hours. Inhaled therapy is preferable to tablets as it means that the drug is delivered directly to the lungs where it works and does not affect the rest of the body. Short-acting beta agonist drugs are used for the relief of symptoms such as wheezing, coughing and breathlessness as well as before situations such as exercise in which the person with asthma knows that symptoms are likely to occur.

bronchodilator drug
A medication used to treat asthma symptoms, also known as a reliever. Bronchodilators work by relaxing the muscles around the airways and making breathing easier.

preventive drug
A medication which reduces the severity of asthma when taken regularly over a prolonged period. Preventive drugs work by turning off the underlying disease process in asthma.

inhaler
A device that delivers asthma medication to the airways. There are several different types of inhalers including the metered dose inhaler and dry powder inhaler.

my experience

I had real difficulty working out how severe my asthma was during bad attacks. My doctor eventually developed a system with me whereby I kept a close eye on the amount of short-acting beta agonist I used. When I end up using it every few hours I go along to my doctor for review and additional treatment. I know that if for any reason I need it more than every hour, I need to call an ambulance.

myth

Asthma can be cured by treatment

fact

Unfortunately, although treatment can lead to excellent control, it can not lead to a 'cure'. However, many people with asthma grow out of it over time, and so the hope is that with long-term treatment asthma can be well controlled until this happens. It is important to note that asthma is a variable disease and can vary in severity over a lifetime.

The amount of short-acting beta agonist used gives an excellent guide to the patient and doctor about the level of asthma control and whether additional treatment is required. In this way it is generally recommended that if a person with asthma uses their short-acting beta agonist most days of the week, they probably also require a regular preventive medication such as an inhaled steroid. Likewise, a person with asthma should be advised that if at any time they need to use their short-acting beta agonist every two to three hours, it is likely they have developed an attack of sufficient severity to warrant going to see their doctor. If a person with asthma gets even worse and has a minimal response to very frequent use of their short-acting beta agonist drug (for example every 30 to 60 minutes), it is a sign that they have a potentially life-threatening attack of asthma and should seek emergency medical care immediately.

A few words of caution are necessary regarding the use of short-acting beta agonists. Because they are so effective there is a tendency for some asthmatic patients to repeatedly take their short-acting beta agonist in the situation of severe asthma, without seeking medical help, reassured by the response they obtain (even if only temporary). This can lead to delay in seeking medical care for a severe attack and put the patient's life at unnecessary risk. Patients should discuss with the doctor how much short-acting beta agonist they can take in an attack before they must call for help.

In treating a person experiencing a severe attack of asthma, short-acting beta agonist therapy may be given through a **nebulizer** driven by oxygen or compressed air. This method of delivery is preferred by many people with asthma due, in part, to the greater relief they obtain with the higher dose that is delivered, and the comfort of the face mask. Although it is common practice for nebulizers to be used in this setting, the same benefit can actually be achieved with five puffs of a short-acting beta agonist via a **metered dose inhaler** (MDI) and **spacer**.

nebulizer

A nebulizer is a device which pumps air through a liquid (in a pot), thereby creating a fine mist of aerosol droplets. If the solution is an asthma medication, the resulting mist can be breathed in by a patient with asthma through a face mask or mouthpiece.

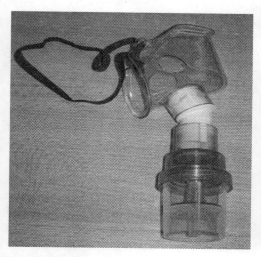

Figure 5.1 A nebulizer.

metered dose inhaler (MDI)

An MDI is the usual device which people with asthma use to deliver their medications. When the canister is pressed it releases the medication as an aerosol, which the patient breathes into their lungs, where it exerts its effect.

 Q **Why is my doctor not keen on me getting a nebulizer to use at home?**

 A The main concern with the use of nebulizers by patients at home is that when used in severe asthma attacks, they may give a false sense of security due to the response to the bigger dose of bronchodilator administered. As a result patients may use their nebulizer repeatedly and delay seeking medical help until their asthma reaches the stage when their life is seriously at risk. This has led many doctors to follow the simple rule that if you need a nebulizer then you need to see a doctor.

spacer

A spacer is a chamber which holds the medication for the person to breathe in. An MDI is inserted in one end of the spacer; the medication is released as an aerosol from the MDI into the spacer; the patient with asthma breathes in the aerosol through a one-way valve at the other end of the spacer.

fact

Contrary to common opinion, the use of an MDI via a spacer is as effective as a nebulizer for delivering short-acting beta agonists in the situation of severe asthma. That is why in some hospital emergency departments or GP clinics doctors use an MDI plus spacer rather than nebulizer therapy. This method is especially preferred for children who may find the nebulizer mask claustrophobic.

Long-acting beta agonist drugs

There is another group of beta agonist drugs called long-acting beta agonists (LABAs), which are also delivered from an inhaler device. LABAs last for at least 12 hours and as a result are normally taken only twice a day. They are prescribed as add-on therapy, recommended in patients whose asthma is not controlled despite inhaled steroid therapy (preventive therapy). The LABAs should not be used as a sole therapy but must be given alongside regular inhaled steroids. One way in which this can be guaranteed is by using a 'combination product' which delivers both an inhaled steroid and a LABA from a single inhaler, thereby giving both preventive and bronchodilator drugs at the same time.

Anticholinergics

Anticholinergic drugs are similar to beta agonist drugs in that they also relax the airway muscles but they are not as effective in asthma as they are in COPD (see page 29). They can be taken from either a combination inhaler device which also administers a beta agonist, or from a separate inhaler. They are normally used in older patients who may also have chronic bronchitis, and are of greater benefit to this age group than to younger asthma sufferers. The other situation in which an anticholinergic drug may be used is in a severe asthma attack which requires nebulizer therapy, and in this case it is given together with a short-acting beta agonist drug.

Oral theophylline

These medications have been used in the treatment of asthma since the 1960s. They are available in tablet form and are normally taken once or twice a day. Improvements in formulation of theophylline tablets have led to slow release preparations which result in steady blood levels throughout the day and night. This has led to an increase in their effectiveness while reducing their tendency to cause side effects. Theophyllines are normally taken as an add-on therapy in a patient whose asthma is not controlled with inhaled steroids and short-acting beta agonist drugs. It can sometimes be difficult to determine the best dose of this medication for a patient and, as a result, the level of this drug in the blood is sometimes measured as a guide. This is especially important if side effects (nausea, vomiting and palpitations) are suspected.

Leukotriene receptor antagonists

A more recent class of medication is the leukotriene receptor antagonist drugs (LTRAs, sometimes called leukotriene modifiers), which have similar effects to those of oral theophylline. Like theophylline, LTRAs probably have some preventive effects as well as having bronchodilator action. The LTRAs are taken in tablet form, normally as an add-on therapy, by patients whose asthma is poorly controlled despite standard therapy. Different from theophylline, they

Q What are the symptoms that suggest that the theophylline dose is too high?

A Theophylline toxicity is suggested by feeling sick and restless, vomiting and a fast heart rate. If a person with asthma on theophylline experiences these symptoms they need to have a blood test to measure the theophylline level as it suggests the dose is too high and needs to be reduced.

Q Are there any situations where LTRAs may be particularly beneficial?

A People with asthma who are sensitive to aspirin may respond well to LTRA therapy. Due to the varying response to the different medications in asthma, a trial of different medications is worthwhile in those with poor control of their asthma.

are normally free from side effects and are especially valuable for those who have difficulty using inhalers, and in those with aspirin (non-steroidal anti-inflammatory drug – NSAID)-induced asthma – an uncommon but serious form of the asthma disease.

Preventive drugs

Preventive therapy acts by turning off or dampening down the underlying disease processes in asthma. Preventive therapy is often referred to as 'anti-inflammatory' because the disease process in asthma is referred to as inflammation. In asthma the underlying inflammation causes a thickening of the airway wall and mucus plugging, and makes the airway muscle 'twitchy' or hyperresponsive.

Inhaled steroids

The regular use of inhaled **steroids** is the most effective preventive treatment available for the long-term management of asthma. Inhaled steroids work by reducing the airway inflammation. Their long-term use leads to an improved quality of life and improved lung function, a reduced frequency of severe attacks and a reduced risk of death. Importantly, inhaled steroids are the only medication which can reduce the risk of a life-threatening attack of asthma leading to a hospital admission or death. This underlies their recommended widespread use in asthma.

There is often concern expressed about the potential adverse side effects of inhaled steroid therapy. In fact, the risk of a patient with asthma who is using inhaled steroid therapy developing these side effects is very small, particularly with the low doses of inhaled steroids that are used to control most people's asthma. However, with

steroids
A group of chemicals that is produced naturally in the body by the adrenal gland. There are many types of steroids that are used for medical purposes. In asthma, steroids are used to reduce the underlying disease process – the inflammation of the airways.

myth
Inhaled steroids should be reserved for adult patients who have severe asthma.

fact
Inhaled steroids are recommended for adult patients with persistent asthma but regardless of severity. The general rule to go by is that if an adult patient with asthma requires their bronchodilator inhaler on most days they also need an inhaled steroid inhaler every day. It is also recommended that inhaled steroids are used in children with moderate and severe persistent asthma, but at a lower dose.

long-term use of high doses of inhaled steroids, together with frequent courses of oral steroids for severe attacks or the taking of steroids by other routes, for example via the skin for eczema, there is a small risk of developing thin bones, stunted growth (in children), adrenal suppression (reducing the production of the hormone cortisol) and cataracts (lens opacities that impair vision).

> **Q** **Will the regular use of inhaled steroids stunt my child's growth?**
>
> **A** In some children, inhaled steroids may cause some impairment of growth. However, 'catch up' growth will occur later. As a result, on average, children with asthma who take regular inhaled steroids will end up with normal height. In fact the major factor impairing growth in children with persistent asthma is the lack of inhaled steroids, due to the adverse effect that uncontrolled asthma has on their general health including growth. As a result, it is recommended that children with persistent asthma take regular inhaled steroids but at the lowest dose necessary to control their asthma.

Inhaled steroids should be started if the patient has symptoms or requires bronchodilator therapy on most days. The frustrating feature of inhaled steroid therapy is that it usually takes a few weeks of treatment before the patient notices real benefit, and continued benefit requires regular long-term use. Unfortunately this means that patients are far less likely to take their inhaled steroids regularly than their inhaled bronchodilator treatment, from which they almost always feel better immediately after its use. Although most patients are encouraged to take their inhaled steroids twice a day, a once-daily regimen is often adequate in a person with mild asthma.

For patients with poorly controlled asthma, one convenient way to take inhaled steroid therapy is

myth
Regular use of inhaled steroids for asthma will mean you will end up looking like a body builder.

fact
The steroids used to treat asthma are completely different from the anabolic steroids used by some body builders and athletes. As a result, there is no risk whatsoever of looking like a body builder. Furthermore, taking steroids from an inhaler means that only very small doses are taken and, as it goes straight down to the airways, almost none is absorbed into the rest of the body.

Q **What is the standard oral steroid regime prescribed for severe asthma?**

A For adults, there is a number of regimes commonly used:
(a) A fixed dose for a defined period, e.g. 40 mg prednisolone for five days;
(b) A decreasing dose regime, e.g. 8, 7, 6, 5, 4, 3, 2, 1 x 5 mg prednisolone tablets;
(c) A variable dose regime in which prednisolone is normally started at 40 mg per day and continued at this dose until definite improvement has been achieved. Prednisolone is then continued at 20 mg per day for the same number of days, i.e. if it takes three days of prednisolone at 40 mg a day for the attack to come right, prednisolone is then taken at 20 mg a day for a further three days.
In children the doses are generally lower and the duration of treatment is shorter than in adults.

by using a combination inhaler which also contains a long-acting beta-agonist. This has a number of potential advantages including improved adherence with the inhaled steroid component as the patient takes the combination inhaler more regularly due to the symptomatic benefit gained from the long-acting beta-agonist component.

Cromones

The cromones are another class of preventive drugs which is given by inhalation. The two drugs in this class are called sodium cromoglycate and nedocromil sodium and these are effective in improving asthma control when taken regularly on a long-term basis. However, their use has been limited as they have less benefit than inhaled steroids and they must be taken four times a day. As a result they are less frequently used, being reserved mainly for specific situations such as before provoked asthma which occurs from stimuli such as exercise and in people who have a strong allergic component to their asthma. They are occasionally used for treating asthma in children.

Oral steroids

Steroid tablets are normally used only for the treatment of severe attacks of asthma. In this situation they are the most effective medication to treat the attack. They are normally taken for one to two weeks in a severe attack and are not continued long term due to the risk of adverse effects.

However, there are some very severe asthma patients who require long-term oral steroids, normally at as low a dose as possible. The prolonged use of oral steroids may cause significant long-term side effects such as thin bones, adrenal suppression, thinning and bruising of the skin, and cataracts, the latter two being largely restricted to older people taking oral steroids. In such patients it is worthwhile having their bone density and adrenal function measured every three to five years.

Other oral anti-inflammatory drugs

There are a number of bronchodilator medications that have some anti-inflammatory effect such as oral theophylline and leukotriene receptor antagonist drugs (see pages 47–8). Both are taken in tablet form on a regular basis which allows the maximum benefit to be obtained.

Allergen immunotherapy

Allergen-specific immunotherapy involves repeated injections of extracts of allergen under the skin. In this way an attempt is made to 'desensitize' the person with asthma to the allergens to which they may be allergic. It is less effective than standard forms of therapy and, because it carries the risk of a life-threatening allergic response, it is not recommended for standard use. Due to this risk, immunotherapy requires close medical supervision and is only used for asthma when other treatments have failed or where a single allergen is especially problematic, for example grass or tree pollen, cat danders.

The benefits of immunotherapy outweigh the risks in some other conditions such as life-threatening bee or wasp venom reactions, where it is the preferred treatment. It is also valuable in treating seasonal allergic rhinitis (hay fever), but as with other conditions, must be conducted in a specialist allergy centre. Sublingual immunotherapy (SLIT), in which the allergen is taken under the tongue, is a new, safer form that is being trialled in mild asthma. In addition, new allergen vaccines with a lower risk of side effects are now in clinical trial.

> **myth**
> In severe asthma attacks oral steroids such as prednisolone always need to be given for a two- to three-week period.

> **fact**
> In severe asthma attacks the length of the course of oral steroids will depend on how severe and how long the attack goes on for. Generally, the earlier that oral steroids are started the shorter the course that is required. Often a short course of a week is fine.

 What is immunotherapy?

Immunotherapy is a treatment designed to reduce the sensitivity of the immune system to allergens; it involves a series of injections of allergen under the skin. Unfortunately, immunotherapy has proven not to be of major benefit in asthma and as there is also a risk of developing serious allergic reactions to the injections, it is not commonly prescribed.

fact

Most severe attacks of asthma are not caused by bacterial infections and as a result do not require antibiotic therapy. In contrast to bacterial infections, viruses ranging from the common cold virus through to influenza are common causes of severe attacks of asthma. However, viruses do not respond to antibiotic therapy. As a general rule, patients with attacks of asthma only require an antibiotic if they have yellow or green phlegm, or discoloured nasal discharge.

Antibiotics

There should be special mention of the use of antibiotics in asthma. Antibiotics treat bacterial infections not viral infections. Bacterial infections rarely provoke attacks of asthma and as a result antibiotics are not routinely used for severe attacks. Viral infections such as the common cold or the flu do commonly cause asthma attacks. Antibiotics are ineffective in this situation as they do not work against viral infections.

As with all rules there are some exceptions, such as in the older person with asthma who has been a smoker and also has chronic bronchitis, in whom an antibiotic may be needed in an attack brought on by a chest infection. Another exception is sinusitis which is commonly due to a bacterial infection and so antibiotics may need to be prescribed. As a result antibiotics would normally be prescribed if there is discoloured phlegm or nasal discharge.

Common drug names (with trade name in brackets)

Bronchodilator drugs

Short-acting beta agonists – inhaled/MDI, dry powder devices, nebulizer solution®

Salbutamol	(Ventolin®, Airomir®)
Terbutaline	(Bricanyl®)
Pirbuterol	(Muxair®)
Procaterol	(Pro-Air®)

Long-acting beta agonists – inhaled/MDI, dry powder devices

Salmeterol	(Severent®, Flovent®)
Formoterol	(Oxis®, Foradil®)

Anticholinergics – short acting – inhaled/MDI, dry powder devices, nebulizer solution
Ipratropium   (Atrovent®)

Theophylline – tablets
Theophylline   (Theodur®, Nuelin®)

Leukotriene receptor antagonists – oral/tablets
Montelukast   (Singulair®)
Zafirlukast   (Accolate®)

Preventive drugs

Steroids – inhaled/MDI, dry powder devices
Beclomethasone   (BDP®, Becotide®,
                                   Becloforte®,
                                   Qvar®)
Budesonide   (Pulmicort®)
Flunisolide   (Bronalide®)
Fluticasone   (Flixotide®)
Mometasone   (Asmanex®)
Triamcinolone   (Azmacort®)

Non-steroids – inhaled/MDI
Sodium cromoglycate   (Intal®)
Nedocromil sodium   (Tilade®)

Combination drugs

Short-acting beta agonist and anticholinergics – inhaled/MDI, nebulizer solution
Salbutamol/Ipratropium   (Combivent®)

Inhaled steroid and long-acting beta agonist – inhaled/MDI, dry powder devices
Fluticasone/Salbutamol   (Seretide, Advair®)
Budesonide/Fomoterol   (Symbicort®)

Stepwise approach

A stepwise approach is recommended in the management of asthma. This involves stepping up treatment as necessary to gain control and stepping down treatment when control has been maintained for a prolonged period (see Figure 5.2). A doctor normally starts treatment at the level at which it is likely that control will be achieved.

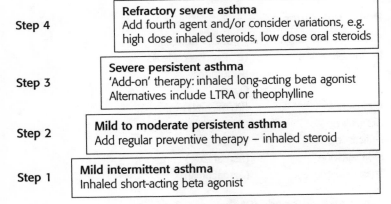

Step 4

Refractory severe asthma
Add fourth agent and/or consider variations, e.g. high dose inhaled steroids, low dose oral steroids

Step 3

Severe persistent asthma
'Add-on' therapy: inhaled long-acting beta agonist
Alternatives include LTRA or theophylline

Step 2

Mild to moderate persistent asthma
Add regular preventive therapy – inhaled steroid

Step 1

Mild intermittent asthma
Inhaled short-acting beta agonist

↑Poor control: step up ↓Prolonged good control: step down

Figure 5.2 Stepwise management, in which patients step up or step down depending on asthma control.

If asthma does not come under good control with standard asthma management then there is often a simple reason, such as the patient not taking the preventive therapy regularly, the patient having difficulty using their inhalers with the correct technique or even that the diagnosis of asthma itself may be incorrect.

Inhaler technique and compliance

The most common reasons for poor asthma control are that patients are either not taking their preventive inhalers regularly or are not using their inhalers correctly.

Technique

It is crucial that patients with asthma learn how to use their inhaler devices correctly, to ensure that the drug gets down into their lungs where it works. The standard device is the MDI (see page 45) in which the patient presses the inhaler canister to release the drug as an aerosol while breathing in at the same time. Even with repeated instruction some patients, particularly the young and elderly, may still have difficulty with co-ordination and need to use another device.

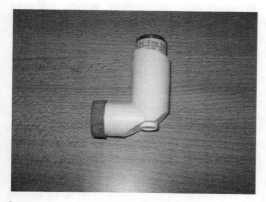

Figure 5.3 A metered dose inhaler (MDI).

How to use an MDI

Remember . . . breathe in slowly to draw the treatment dose right down.

1 Shake the inhaler.
2 Sit upright and hold your chin up.
3 Breathe out with a sigh.

4 Hold the inhaler upright and close your lips around the mouthpiece.

5 As you begin to breathe in *slowly* and *deeply*, press the inhaler once.

6 Hold your breath for about five to ten seconds.

7 Breathe out slowly and gently through your nose.

8 After a minute, repeat these steps for further doses.

9 Rinse your mouth and gargle after using a steroid inhaler.

dry powder inhaler
A device that automatically releases a medication as a dry powder when a patient breathes in through the mouthpiece. Such devices are also referred to as 'breath actuated inhalers'.

Alternative dry powder devices that are simpler to use have been produced in order to avoid the difficulties of using an MDI. These **dry powder inhalers** are also called 'breath actuated inhalers' as they are activated by the patient breathing in, thereby not requiring co-ordination in their use. The most commonly used dry powder devices are the Turbuhaler® and the Accuhaler®, (see Figure 5.4).

Dry powder devices are particularly useful for those patients who have difficulty operating an MDI, such as children and older people. Each device has its own features and if patients do prefer these then, as for MDI's, they should receive instructions from their health professional on how to operate the device and how to optimally inhale the drug it administers. Most drugs available as MDI's are also available as dry powder devices.

Spacer devices are holding chambers which are used with a metered dose inhaler (MDI) (see page 45). The MDI is inserted into the spacer, so that when it is pressed it releases the drug aerosol into the chamber which the patient then breathes

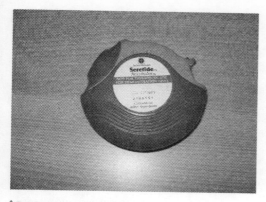

| Figure 5.4 An accuhaler.

in through a one-way valve. This technique does not require co-ordination between pressing and breathing and results in better inhalation of the drug into the lungs. It is not convenient to carry a spacer around due to its size and so it is normally reserved for use at home, primarily with inhaled steroids which need to be taken only once or twice a day. The other situation when a spacer is used is during a severe attack of asthma, in which five puffs of a short-acting beta agonist from an MDI through a spacer results in a similar benefit as a standard dose from a nebulizer.

Q **Is there a problem with the use of MDIs containing CFCs?**

A Until recently MDIs have contained **chlorofluorocarbons (CFCs)** as propellants which have enabled the active drug to be dispersed as an aerosol. However, there is concern that CFCs are responsible for depletion of the earth's ozone layer and even though asthma medications only contribute to around 1 per cent of all CFCs released into the atmosphere, they are being phased out. They are being replaced by

chlorofluoro-carbons (CFCs)
The propellants used in MDIs which are damaging to the ozone layer.

hydrofluoro-carbons (HFAs)
The propellants that have replaced CFCs in MDIs due to their lack of harmful effects on the ozone layer.

either MDIs including **hydrofluorocarbons (HFAs)** (rather than CFCs) which do not damage the ozone layer, or dry powder devices which do not require an aerosol propellant. The major sources of emissions of CFCs into the atmosphere are fridges, air conditioning units and spray cans.

How to use an MDI with a spacer

1 Shake the inhaler.
2 Fit the inhaler into the spacer opening.
3 Press the inhaler once only.
4 Breathe in *slowly* and *deeply* through the spacer mouthpiece.
5 Hold your breath for five to ten seconds OR, if breathless, take two to three normal breaths, keeping the spacer in your mouth all the time.
6 Repeat these steps for further doses.
7 Once a month, wash your spacer with warm water and washing-up liquid and leave to dry in the air.

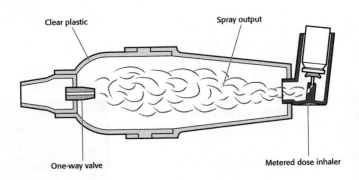

Clear plastic

Spray output

One-way valve

Metered dose inhaler

Figure 5.5 MDI with spacer.

Compliance

In asthma, **compliance** or **concordance** with taking inhaled steroid medications regularly as prescribed by a doctor is a particular problem. Unlike bronchodilator medications, patients feel no immediate benefit as inhaled steroids work by turning off the asthma process over time, rather than by relaxing the muscles and giving immediate relief of symptoms. Another difference is that the best results with inhaled steroids occur with regular use even when the patient with asthma is well and has few symptoms. However, if patients are not troubled by symptoms they often do not take the inhaled steriods due to feeling that they are not required. This may go some way towards explaining why people with asthma may take on average only half the inhaled steroid medication they are prescribed.

Compliance is closely related to the simplicity of the regime and the number of doses taken per day. It is for this reason that the recommended use of inhaled steroids has decreased from four times daily in the 1980s to twice daily in the 1990s, and that inhaled steroids which can be used once a day are currently being developed.

compliance

The extent to which a person's behaviour, in terms of taking medication or making lifestyle changes, coincides with the advice from a doctor. It assumes that a correct diagnosis has been made, that the doctor's advice is appropriate and that the patient is able to follow the advice.

concordance

The extent to which an agreed plan is followed by the patient. In contrast to compliance, concordance shows respect for the aims of both the doctor and the patient and means that there has been a negotiated agreement between the two.

Q Do I need to take my inhalers when I feel well?

A Yes (and no). You should take your preventive inhaler (such as inhaled steroid) even when you are well, as this ensures that your asthma remains under good control. In contrast, you do not need to take your reliever inhaler (such as a short-acting beta agonist) if you are not experiencing symptoms. Reliever medications need only be taken to relieve symptoms should they occur. If a patient with asthma uses this recommended approach, the amount of reliever inhaler that they take can be used as a guide to how bad their asthma is at any one time.

Q Do I have to take my inhaled steroid twice a day?

A Although it is recommended that inhaled steroids are taken twice a day, for many patients with mild asthma and infrequent attacks the same total dose taken once a day is an acceptable alternative. This change would normally be undertaken only after discussion with a doctor or nurse.

Another approach has been the incorporation of inhaled steroids with a long-acting beta agonist drug (LABA) within the same 'combination' inhaler. This combination inhaler represents a simple and convenient treatment that not only leads to improved compliance with inhaled steroids but also ensures that the LABA is not taken as sole therapy.

Useful treatment tips

Here is a number of handy tips which a person with asthma might follow to ensure that they get the best possible results from their medications:

- ✧ Ask your doctor, nurse or pharmacist about the role of each of your medications. Ask for written instructions on when and how to use each one, as part of your written action plan.
- ✧ Know the side effects of your medication so you understand what is and isn't normal. If you have any concerns about your medications, talk to your doctor, nurse or pharmacist.
- ✧ If you have been prescribed a preventive medication, keep taking it even when you feel well. It needs to be taken regularly and long term to work effectively.
- ✧ Ask your doctor or nurse if your medication regime can be simplified. One way is to have the same type of inhaler device for your different medications, so you don't have to get used to several kinds.
- ✧ Ask your doctor or nurse to give you an inhaler device that you feel comfortable with. There are special types to help you if you have trouble co-ordinating the 'press and breathe' kind.

✧ Even the best medication will only work if you take it correctly. Ask your doctor, nurse or pharmacist to check your inhaler technique regularly.

✧ Create memory aids for yourself, like always taking your asthma medication when you brush your teeth in the morning and evening.

✧ Keep a record of your reliever medication purchases so you know how often you need to get more and can inform your doctor at your check-ups.

my experience

I could never remember to take my preventive inhaler as I was always in a rush in the morning and often forgot at night. Whenever I woke at night or got worse I promised myself that I would remember to take my inhalers more regularly – but I didn't. When my doctor asked me whether I took my inhalers regularly and I mentioned my difficulties, she suggested that I put my preventive inhaler by my toothbrush and use it before I cleaned my teeth morning and night, (which I am good at remembering) – then gargle and rinse my mouth out. This worked really well and it was quite nice to get rid of the taste and within a few weeks my asthma was getting under far better control. The other reminder options she suggested were putting my preventive inhaler by my bed to take when I got in or out of bed or taking it to work to take when I arrived in the morning and left in the evening.

Severe attacks

Treatment

The standard treatment for severe attacks of asthma is the repeated use of high doses of inhaled short-acting beta agonists, oral steroids, oxygen and close medical practitioner review. It is preferable that this treatment is given in the setting of a doctor's surgery or hospital emergency department to ensure that the response to treatment can be monitored and to see if there is a need for hospital admission. However, before any medical review, the decision making is in the hands of the patient and there are a few principles that are useful to follow.

Patients should have written guidelines on when to seek medical help. They should be encouraged to use their inhaled short-acting beta agonist as often as needed in a severe attack while medical help is being sought. In addition to treating the severe attack, the frequency of and response to their beta agonist allows the patient to decide how severe their asthma is. There is commonly a reluctance for patients to seek medical assistance when experiencing severe asthma attacks as they hope that the attack will eventually settle. However, patients should understand that the earlier they seek medical help and receive oral steroids during a severe attack, the quicker their ashtma will improve. They will also require a shorter course of oral steroid therapy, and are less likely to be admitted to hospital.

Non-drug based approaches

Primary prevention

primary prevention
Intervention made before any evidence of disease to prevent the disease from developing.

The most effective measures to reduce the risk of an infant developing asthma is both to breastfeed and to make sure that there is no exposure to tobacco smoke. Parents (and parents to be), who smoke should know of the many health risks that smoking causes their children, including asthma, and should be offered advice and support to stop smoking. Despite the strong relationship between exposure to allergens and asthma, the results of allergen avoidance programmes have been disappointing and as a result they cannot be strongly recommended at this stage.

Secondary prevention

There are a number of measures that a person with asthma might consider to reduce its impact. While any benefit may well be variable and difficult to predict, it should be considered.

Avoiding allergens is one approach although there has been little evidence of major benefit. Approaches have focused on either reducing exposure to the common major allergens such as house-dust mite, cat, dog and cockroach allergens, or to focus on a specific allergen that is recognized by the patient's personal experience or through skin prick testing. Below is a checklist of measures that might be tried in the case of the common allergens:

House-dust mite

✧ Use protective coverings on pillows and mattresses
✧ Wash bedding regularly at 55–60°C
✧ Ensure the house is ventilated, and reduce any dampness.

Pets

✧ Do not get a pet if you haven't already got one
✧ Exclude pets from bedrooms
✧ Vacuum regularly.

Cockroaches

✧ Eradicate cockroaches with insecticides
✧ Seal cracks in floors and ceilings
✧ Remove sources of food, and reduce any dampness.

secondary prevention
Intervention made after the onset of disease to reduce its impact.

Q What can I do to improve my home environment in general?

A It is important that your home is well ventilated, dry and kept clean, particularly the floors. Wood, tile or linoleum flooring is better than fitted textile carpeting, which tends to collect a lot of dust and allergens. Do not keep furry animals or birds, even if you are not specifically allergic to them, as they will lead to an increase in the amount of house dust. Try to avoid strong perfumes, aftershave, deodorants and fragrant flowers inside the house, as these are all possible triggers of asthma. Do not allow anyone to smoke indoors.

Mould

✧ Ensure the house is ventilated
✧ Reduce any dampness
✧ Remove mould using solution containing
   5 per cent ammonia.

When asthma is triggered by occupational exposures such as chemicals or other sensitizing agents, the person must remove themselves from the sources of exposure in the workplace (see Chapter 7).

The evidence for the benefits of giving up smoking is substantial, not only to reduce asthma severity but also to reduce the risk of developing other serious disorders later in life such as lung cancer, heart attacks and strokes. In patients with asthma, smoking also decreases the effectiveness of inhaled steroids. Details of methods to help stop smoking are provided in Chapter 7.

Exercise does not appear to reduce asthma severity but does lead to improved fitness which may be of real benefit to a person with asthma. As a result, regular exercise is recommended as part of a general approach to improve wellbeing in a person with asthma.

Currently there is not enough evidence to support the use of acupuncture, air ionizers, homeopathy, hypnosis or breathing exercises such as yoga and Buteyko. This does not mean that such measures would not be helpful; rather, it means that no clear recommendation can be made at this stage due to the lack of evidence to prove they help. If patients do wish to try these complementary medical therapies then they should be in addition to rather than instead of recommended drug therapy.

CHAPTER

6

Guided self-management – putting it all together

The approach

The approach of **guided self-management** was developed as clinicians tried to design methods by which they could put together all the different aspects of asthma management and deliver better asthma care. It is where patients with asthma learn to recognize unstable or deteriorating asthma early on and, by following written guidelines, know when it is necessary to adjust treatment or get medical assistance.

These are five basic principles of guided self-management in asthma:

1 The need for patients to assess the severity of their asthma, by recognizing key symptoms and by measuring peak flow.
2 The use of regular inhaled steroids and 'as required' short-acting beta agonists for the long-term treatment of asthma.

> **guided self-management**
> Management approach in which patients control their own condition with guidance from the health care professional.

Q **Is guided self-management used with any medical disorders other than asthma?**

A Yes, this approach is well established in diabetes in which patients often have difficulty telling how well their diabetes is controlled by how well they feel. To overcome this difficulty people with diabetes are trained to measure their blood sugar levels on a regular basis. They then refer to written guidelines to work out how much insulin they should take.

3 The use of oral steroids, high dose inhaled short-acting beta agonists, and medical care for severe attacks.

4 The combination of self-assessment and self-management.

5 The need for written guidelines for both long-term treatment and the treatment of severe attacks.

Asthma action plans

The following table shows the standard **asthma action plan** based on the above principles. The first two stages provide guidelines for the regular long-term treatment of asthma. The third and fourth stages provide guidelines for the patient to recognize the development of severe asthma and to start more intensive treatment to try to avoid a life-threatening attack.

Table 2 Prototype asthma action plan: What to do and when

Stage	Peak flow	Symptoms	Action
1	>80% best	Intermittent/few	Continue regular inhaled steroids (consider reduction if patient is well for several months) and inhaled beta agonist as required for relief of symptoms
2	<80% best	Waking at night with asthma; increasing beta agonist use	Start inhaled steroid treatment or increase the dose
3	<60–70% best	Increasing breathlessness or using beta agonist 2–3 times hourly	Start oral steroids and contact a doctor
4	<40–50% best	Severe attack of asthma, poor response to beta agonist	Call an emergency doctor or ambulance urgently

At all stages, take inhaled beta agonist for relief of symptoms

The use of the written action plans is now considered to represent 'optimal management' which can achieve the best outcomes in asthma. This recommendation is based on research which has shown that use of the plans leads to a marked improvement in asthma control and, in particular, a reduction in severe attacks leading to hospital admissions. The way in which a patient with asthma uses an action plan in a progressively worsening attack of asthma is shown in Figure 6.1 on page 68.

Several adult asthma self-management plans are available on-line. The following websites have asthma plans freely downloadable:

◇ The Asthma UK action plan is available at www.asthma.org.uk/about/control.php
◇ The New Zealand Asthma and Respiratory Foundation asthma action plan is available at www.asthmanz.co.nz (Figure 6.2, page 69)
◇ The Australian National Asthma Campaign plan is available at www.nationalasthma.org.au/publications/action/html/adults.html
◇ Asthma self-management, Interactive Euro Health at www.interactive.eurohealth.com/asthma.html

asthma action plan
A written plan that provides patients with guidelines for the assessment and management of asthma.

Q What do I do if I have a severe attack and cannot find my peak flow meter?

A If you do not have a peak flow meter handy it is fine to simply follow the symptom part of the action plan. The amount of inhaled bronchodilator you need to relieve your symptoms is an excellent guide to tell you how bad you are and what other treatment you require.

Individual requirements

No single plan is likely to be suitable for every patient as their requirements may vary considerably. Certain features may need to be varied, depending on the needs and preferences of the patient for whom the plan is developed.

myth
A standard action plan can be used by all patients.

fact
The standard action plan may have to be significantly modified by a doctor so that it meets the needs and preferences of individual patients.

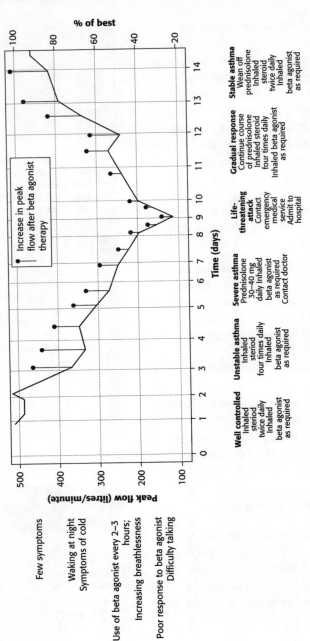

Figure 6.1 Use of a self-management plan in a patient with deteriorating asthma. In this example, an asthma attack develops over one week. The patient recognizes stages of worsening asthma by the development of key symptoms and institutes changes in management according to predetermined written guidelines.

Asthma self-management plan instructions

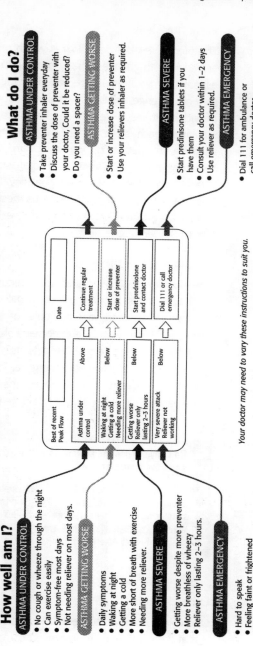

Figure 6.2 The New Zealand Asthma and Respiratory Foundation asthma action plan.

myth

Many patients find action plans too difficult and get into trouble if they try to use them.

fact

Research has shown that most patients do not have any difficulty becoming familiar with their action plan and using it effectively. However, it does require the doctor or nurse being flexible in making sure that the plans meet the needs and preferences of the patient. It is certainly a situation where 'one size does not fit all'.

Peak flow levels

The precise level of peak flow at which patients are advised to change therapy or seek medical assistance may need to be varied for different patients. A range of peak flow values is normally provided at each level for the patient to recognize each stage of asthma severity. For example, the patient recognizes severe asthma requiring medical review and oral steroids (Stage 3 on Table 2), when the peak flow falls to less than 70 per cent of previous best, and should have taken action before the peak flow falls to 60 per cent of best.

Simplifying the plan

One way to simplify the plan is to reduce the number of stages. For example, some patients do not want to have to vary the dose of inhaled steroid; for these patients, a three-stage plan may be all that they need. Some other patients may just want to know when to seek emergency medical care in the situation of a severe asthma attack. These patients can use a simple two-stage plan.

Q Do I have to use the Asthma UK action plan or can I use a simpler plan?

A Yes (and no). While the Asthma UK action plan is strongly recommended, it may be that a different, simpler version better suits your needs. Probably the simplest plan available is a written instruction on when to seek emergency medical care in a severe attack.

Other benefits

One of the unexpected benefits of action plans is that their use leads to improved compliance.

This is because patients are more likely to realize when their asthma is not well controlled and, as a result, are more motivated to take their regular preventive therapy. It has been shown that by using a plan, average compliance improves by about 50 per cent. It is likely that this greater level of compliance is the main reason for improvement in patients who use plans.

Tailoring the recommendations

Certain people with asthma may benefit more than others from asthma plans. The greatest benefit is likely to be obtained in patients with chronic severe asthma, while patients with mild asthma are unlikely to benefit to any great extent from their regular use. The following is a guide for the use of self-management plans according to asthma severity.

Mild asthma

In mild asthma, an asthma diary which records the symptoms and peak flow is used initially to educate the patient to recognize changes in asthma severity, to help the doctor identify those patients who have difficulty recognizing unstable asthma, to work out the 'best' peak flow values for each individual, and to monitor a patient's response to preventive therapy. Following this initial period, a two-stage action plan can be developed which provides simple written instructions as to when to seek medical help in the case of a severe asthma attack. A more detailed self-management plan is not recommended, as it is unlikely to lead to a major improvement in asthma control.

Q **What do I do if my asthma plan says I'm fine but I feel as if I'm in trouble with severe asthma?**

A In this situation, seek medical assistance. The plan is just a guide to assist you and if you feel bad you should get medical help, whatever the plan says.

fact

For patients with mild asthma, after a period of 'getting to know your asthma', with regular monitoring, it is not necessary to measure your peak flow and refer to your action plan every day. For such patients it is better to follow the plan closely with frequent peak flow recordings when asthma is poorly controlled as this is when the guidelines are likely to be most helpful.

Moderate asthma

In patients with moderate asthma, a similar period of assessment is recommended for the same reasons as in mild asthma, and to allow for the development of a more detailed three-stage action plan. The amount of detail included will depend on the requirements of the patient and the degree of medical supervision that is deemed to be necessary. Patients should use the plan preferentially during periods of unstable asthma rather than during periods of good control.

High-risk asthma

For patients with high-risk asthma, such as those with a recent hospital admission, regular peak flow monitoring and recording of symptoms in association with an action plan is recommended, together with intensive medical and nursing supervision.

Q For which patients with asthma is it advisable to follow the action plan most of the time?

A It is recommended that patients who have a poor perception of their asthma (i.e. have difficulty knowing when their asthma is worse), brittle asthma (i.e. have unstable asthma with wide fluctuations of their peak flow) or severe asthma (i.e. frequent severe attacks requiring hospital admission) should monitor their asthma closely using their action plan.

Finally, it should be said that such plans do not necessarily need to be implemented by a doctor. Primary responsibility for the instruction of this system can also be undertaken by a nurse, working in partnership with a doctor. Whatever plan is employed, it needs to reflect the medical practice, resources and health care system of the community in which it is introduced and must be tailored to meet the specific needs of individual patients.

> **Q** **Is there any additional component to the guided self-management system that can be helpful for people with the most severe asthma who frequently end up in hospital?**
>
> **A** There is a system pioneered in Edinburgh in which an ambulance and hospital database is kept of the most severe people with asthma who have required frequent hospital and/or ICU (Intensive Care Unit) admission. The ambulance service is aware that they should be afforded the highest priority when they call for help and, likewise, the hospital ensures that an 'open door' admission policy is followed. Similar systems have been adopted in other districts in the United Kingdom and elsewhere.

my experience

When my doctor first showed me the asthma action plan it looked complicated and I thought I would never be able to use it properly. However it turned out to be really easy. I don't normally use it when I'm well, but when my asthma starts to get worse and I start waking at night with symptoms, I get the plan out and start measuring my peak flow, and note how much bronchodilator inhaler I use. The plan says that for worsening asthma I should double my inhaled steroids – actually, when I have been well for a period, I often stop taking my inhaled steroids and so I suppose that is why I have got worse. I go back on my inhaled steroids and my asthma usually is okay within a few days. If I get worse despite this and I need my bronchodilator inhaler every few hours, my peak flow has usually fallen to around 300 compared with my best values of around 500. At this stage I start my prednisolone tablets myself and give my doctor a call. We normally work out between us how long to carry on with the prednisolone tablets. I know that if I get worse despite these actions, I should get emergency medical help by calling an ambulance, but fortunately this hasn't been necessary so far.

CHAPTER

7

Important special issues

Pregnancy

During pregnancy the severity of asthma often changes and patients may require close follow up and adjustment of medications. However, it is not possible to predict what effect pregnancy might have on a woman's asthma. When women with asthma become pregnant, about one-third will notice an improvement in their asthma, one-third a worsening and in one-third there will be no real difference.

The key to a good outcome for both the mother and baby is to make sure that there is good asthma control throughout the pregnancy. This means that there should be regular treatment with inhaled steroids at the lowest dose to maintain good control and inhaled short-acting beta agonist therapy when required to relieve any asthmatic symptoms. The use of inhaled steroids in pregnancy has been extensively investigated and shown to be safe to both mother and baby.

The two factors that are likely to increase the risk of stunted growth of a baby are maternal smoking and unstable asthma, through causing a reduction in the supply of oxygen to the developing baby. If you want to give your baby the best start in life you should take extra care with your asthma when pregnant and make sure that neither you nor your partner smoke (or anyone else living in your household).

Another situation in which hormonal change may influence asthma in a woman is during her menstrual cycle. About one in three women with asthma develops a worsening of her asthma in the week prior to her menstrual period – this is called **pre-menstrual asthma**. This worsening can usually be controlled by an increase in standard therapy; however, for some women it may be severe and represent a major management problem. Unfortunately there is no hormonal therapy that has been shown to be effective for pre-menstrual asthma.

It is worthwhile discussing pre-menstrual asthma with your doctor to make sure you are taking 'optimal' treatment and there are no other complicating factors. For example, it may be that aspirin or similar medications (called non-steroidal anti-inflammatory drugs, such as nurofen and ponstan) which are commonly used for period pain may contribute to unstable asthma. It is known that these pain relief medications can provoke asthma in susceptible people and so paracetamol may be a better medication to take in this instance.

Q **Can I breastfeed if I am taking asthma medications?**

A Yes, inhaled asthma medications will not affect your baby when you breastfeed as they do not enter the breast milk. There is a number of health advantages in breastfeeding, including a reduced risk of your baby developing allergies such as asthma.

pre-menstrual asthma
A cyclical worsening of asthma control in the week prior to the menstrual period.

Infants and young children

myth

Recurrent coughing at night means a child has asthma.

fact

Recurrent coughing at night, without other problems such as wheezing or breathlessness at night or at other times, is unlikely to be due to asthma. The symptoms are unlikely to respond to asthma medications.

It can be difficult to make a diagnosis of asthma in children under five years of age. In children, repeated episodes of coughing with wheezing, often with shortness of breath, suggest asthma. However, a child having a recurrent cough alone is unlikely to be suffering from asthma and, therefore, is unlikely to respond to standard asthma treatment.

In infants under the age of two years, episodes of wheezing are common, particularly in boys. The wheezing is usually due to a viral respiratory tract infection and simply requires an inhaled bronchodilator if the infant is in distress. Most infants with this type of early wheezing grow out of this problem by the time they are five. Recent clinical trials suggest that leukotriene receptor antagonists for example may also be useful in virus induced wheezing.

In young children up to the age of five, several different patterns of illness occur. Most have infrequent episodes of asthma, lasting about a week every few months or so. These are usually triggered by a viral respiratory tract infection and simply require treatment with an inhaled bronchodilator at the time and a short course of oral steroids if the attack is severe enough to lead to a hospital admission. However, if the episodes are more frequent, the child may require regular preventive treatment such as low dose inhaled steroids in addition to the use of an inhaled bronchodilator when required. One in ten young children who have asthma experiences symptoms on most days in addition to experiencing attacks, and these children also require regular preventive treatment and close monitoring by their doctors.

myth

Action plans are only of benefit to adults with asthma and not children.

fact

The basic principles of asthma management are the same for children aged over five years as they are for adults. This includes action plans. For example, all children with asthma should have written guidelines advising when they need to obtain medical care when experiencing severe asthma.

In children over the age of five years, the assessment and management of asthma is essentially the same as for adults. However, there are some differences, including the use of generally lower doses of medication, such as inhaled steroids, and peak flow meters are not used as much.

In young children and infants there is increasing use of inhaled medications through different inhaler devices. For children under the age of five years, a standard MDI is usually used through a spacer attached to either a face mask or mouthpiece. Children over the age of five years can normally use any of the different inhaler devices that are used by adults, depending on what is preferred. Home nebulizers are not generally recommended for use in infants and young children as they are expensive, time-consuming to use and require maintenance. As a result, nebulizers would be used only when a child with severe asthma cannot master the technique of using the MDI and spacer despite parental training and assistance.

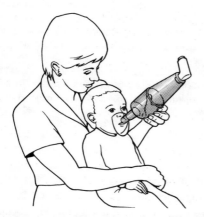

Figure 7.1 A mother giving her young child asthma medication from an MDI and spacer.

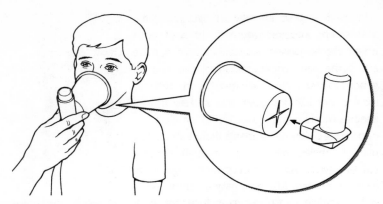

Figure 7.2 An MDI can be used through a plastic cup as an alternative to a spacer.

myth
My three-year-old who has asthma will need to take oral medications as he cannot use inhalers.

fact
It is possible for almost all parents to deliver the medications required in asthma to young children including babies and infants. In the first three years of a child's life this is normally from an MDI through a spacer with a face mask. An alternative to a face mask is a plastic cup with a hole cut in the bottom for the MDI to deliver the drug. These methods do not require co-ordination and can be used to deliver a range of treatments. Between the ages of three and five years, the child may use a normal mouthpiece rather than a face mask connected to the spacer. Parents may still be needed to help deliver the treatment at this age. From the age of five years children should be able to use most inhaler devices as long as they receive training, encouragement and supervision. The reason for preferring inhaled rather than oral medication is that it delivers a high dose to the lungs where it is needed, and less medication goes to the rest of the body.

A related issue is the care of the child with asthma when at school. Many schools have now developed policies for the supervision of children with asthma. This normally means that every student with asthma attending the school has a written record of their usual medications and the actions the teacher should take in the event of an attack. The school should also have standard medications (bronchodilator inhalers) and equipment (such as a spacer device) available in their first-aid kit so that an asthma attack can be managed on site. This is particularly important for school camps, for which supervisors who are competent in acute asthma management should be responsible for the asthma first-aid kit. As a rule, schools should encourage exercise for all students with asthma.

Exercise and sport

Exercise provokes asthma symptoms in most people with asthma. This is called exercise-induced asthma and occurs because there is an increase in both the rate and depth of breathing when someone exercises. This leads to a drying and cooling of the airways, particularly when exercising in cold, dry air. This drying is an irritant to the airways causing the twitchy muscles to go into spasm which in turn causes airways to narrow. The pattern of exercise which is most likely to provoke asthma is six to eight minutes of high intensity exercise, with asthma progressively worsening for 10–15 minutes after the exercise stops. This explains why a person with asthma can often 'run through' their asthma if they exercise beyond eight minutes without stopping.

Q **I've always been told that exercise is good for you, so why can it cause asthma symptoms?**

A Normally, the airways are moist and warm, but during exercise they are exposed to large amounts of dry, cool air as you breathe more rapidly and deeply. This can irritate the already sensitive lining of the airways and cause asthma symptoms or trigger a more severe asthma attack, particularly if your asthma is not well controlled.

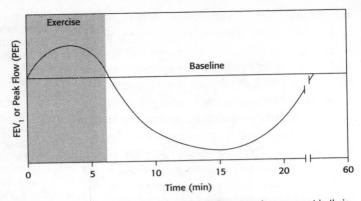

Figure 7.3 A person with asthma usually experiences an improvement in their lung function (FEV₁ or PEF) when they begin exercising. However, if the person stops exercising after about five minutes, their lung function gets worse as they experience a worsening in their asthma. This is called exercise-induced asthma.

If a person is limited by asthma which is induced by exercise, it is a sign that their asthma is not adequately controlled, and that they need an increase in preventive therapy. This is the same as a person who has disturbed sleep due to their asthma, or finds that their asthma is provoked by different irritants in their everyday life. So, as asthma comes under better control one of the first things they will notice is that they can exercise more freely and are not as affected by their asthma in other situations as well.

There is a number of drug and non-drug approaches that may be used to reduce the risk of developing exercise-induced asthma. One option is to do a series of warm-up exercises, such as jogging, for 10–15 minutes before doing any strenuous exercise. This 'acclimatizes' the airways to the effects of exercise. Another option is to ensure that when a person with asthma stops exercising, they should not go into a warm, humid room but rather stay in the environment in which they have exercised for a period of time to 'declimatize'.

myth
The only way to prevent exercise-induced asthma is to take medications before exercising.

fact
While asthma medications are very effective in preventing exercise-induced asthma, warm-up exercises are also helpful and should form part of the routine of a person with asthma before they exercise.

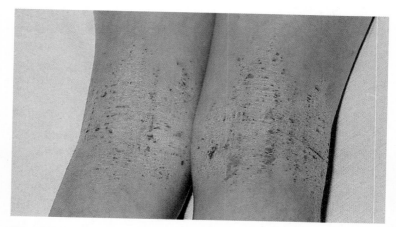

Colour Plate 1
Eczema on the back of a child's legs.

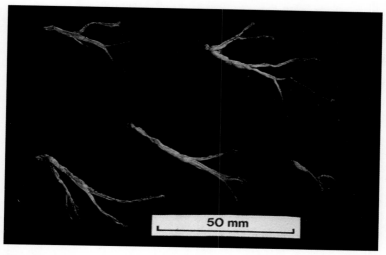

50 mm

Colour Plate 2
Mucus casts from airways coughed up by a person with asthma.

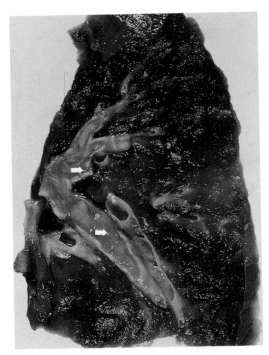

Colour Plate 3
Section of a lung from a patient who died from asthma, showing the occlusion of airways by mucus (arrows).

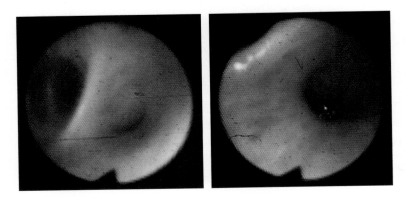

Colour Plate 4
The airways of (left) a healthy person and (right) a person with asthma. The redness and swelling of the airways in asthma is evident.

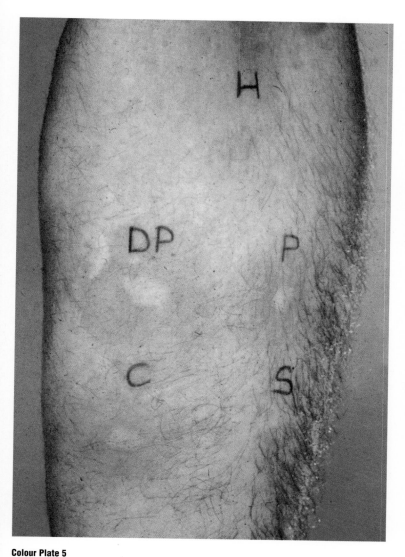

Colour Plate 5
Skin prick tests for common allergies. Strong responses to house dust mite (DP), grass pollen (P), cat dander (C), and positive control (H) are present.

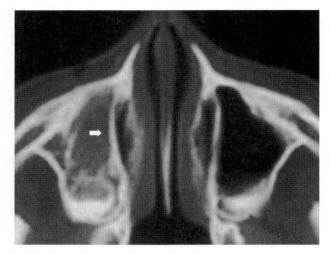

Colour Plate 6
CT scan of sinusitis in which the infected mucus is evident, filling the right nasal cavity (arrow).

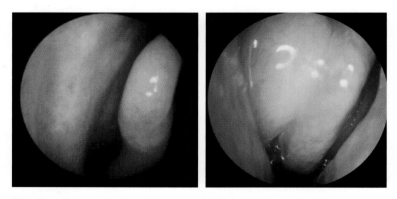

Colour Plate 7
A normal nasal passage (left) and a nasal polyp blocking the nasal passage in a person with asthma (right).

The simplest drug approach is to use a few puffs of short-acting beta agonist prior to exercise. Not only is a short-acting beta agonist very effective in preventing exercise-induced asthma from occurring, it can also be taken if the person with asthma gets symptoms during or after exercise. There are a number of other drugs which can be taken prior to exercise, such as other inhaled bronchodilators, including a long-acting beta agonist or an anticholinergic agent, or a preventive inhaler such as a cromone or leukotriene receptor antagonist.

In terms of sports, swimming is considered the best exercise for people with asthma as it is less likely to provoke an attack due to the air breathed in being warm and humid. In children, swimming can lead to better asthma control, although it may be necessary to try different swimming pools to find the one that suits the child best, often depending on whether the pool uses chlorine, bromine or other cleansing agents.

Elite athletes with asthma need to be aware of the regulations regarding medication use. While different sports have their own specific rules, the standard regulations are those prescribed by the World Anti-doping Agency. These indicate that inhaled steroids, inhaled cromoglycate, inhaled beta agonists (including the long-acting beta agonists salmeterol and formoterol, but not fenoterol, adrenaline or isoprenaline) and oral theophyllines are permitted with a prior medical declaration through an abbreviated therapeutic use exemption. The use of oral steroids for severe attacks is more restrictive, requiring a more detailed exemption. As a general rule, any sports person with asthma competing at a national level or above should be aware of the relevant regulatory requirements and

Q Are some kinds of physical activities more suitable for people with asthma than others?

A Aerobics is a good activity, as it allows you to train at varying intensities. Indoor swimming is also a good exercise, because it takes place at a controlled temperature and in a humid environment. Other types of exercise, such as running, are more likely to provoke asthma. Whatever you do, make sure you warm up first, because this will reduce the likelihood of getting exercise-induced asthma.

myth
People with asthma should not exercise.

fact
It is important that people with asthma exercise regularly to get the general health benefits as well as making sure they overcome their asthma rather than let asthma limit their activities. Examples of elite sports people that have not let their asthma affect their sporting success include Paula Radcliffe (marathon runner), Adrian Moorhouse and Mark Spits (swimmers), Paul Scholes (footballer), and Jackie Joyner-Kersee (track athlete).

occupational asthma
Asthma that develops as a direct result of repeated exposure to substances in the workplace such as fumes or dusts.

notify their national sporting organization of their medication use. Remember: asthma should not be a barrier to an active life. There are many international sports personalities who have become elite in their sport despite having asthma.

Occupational asthma

Asthma may develop as a direct consequence of repeated exposure to substances in the workplace. There are hundreds of different substances that can cause **occupational asthma**, but the main jobs in which occupational asthma have been reported are listed below.

✧ Spray-painters
✧ Sawmill workers or carpenters
✧ Bakers
✧ Smelter workers
✧ Electronics workers
✧ Pharmaceutical industry workers.

The key clues to recognizing occupational asthma is someone developing asthma for the first time as an adult (or someone whose asthma gets a lot worse in adult life) and who experiences improvements in their asthma at weekends and holiday periods. The characteristic pattern is that asthma symptoms gradually develop and worsen months to years after starting work in a particular job. Initially the symptoms may occur only with exposure to the substance in the workplace but, with time, the asthma will occur in other situations (such as with exercise, cold air) similar to other people with asthma. There is a number of other clues that may alert the person with asthma or their doctor to the significance of work exposure in their illness such as:

- Previously no asthma or mild asthma
- Other workers also develop asthma
- Occupation known to be associated with asthma
- Symptoms provoked by exposure to substances at work
- Symptoms worse in the evening or at night after heavy exposure
- Improvement at weekends or on holiday
- Associated symptoms of dermatitis and rhinitis.

It can be difficult to definitely decide if a person has occupational asthma and it may require a period of daily peak flow monitoring (see Figure 7.4) and laboratory tests. It is crucial, however, that the diagnosis of occupational asthma is made with certainty as this means that the person should be removed from any subsequent workplace exposure. The reason for this is that it represents the only chance that the worker has of totally recovering from their asthma. On the other hand, if the worker remains in the workplace with on-going exposure, it is likely they will develop more severe asthma that responds poorly to treatment even after the eventual removal from the occupational exposure that caused the asthma in the first place.

There is another form of occupational wheezing called **reactive airways dysfunction syndrome (RADS)**. This differs from occupational asthma in that it results from one heavy occupational exposure to an irritant substance, such as a chlorine leak. High profile examples include people exposed to fumes from the Bhopal tragedy in India and fire-fighters at the World Trade Center in New York.

Q How is occupational asthma diagnosed?

A Occupational asthma should be suspected in any person who develops asthma for the first time as an adult or whose asthma gets a lot worse in adult life. Regrettably, research indicates that doctors often do not consider this possibility. As a result, it is often left to the patient to raise this issue with their doctor if they suspect this to be the case. The diagnosis is usually confirmed by a characteristic pattern of symptoms and peak flow recordings at work and periods away from work (see Figure 7.4, page 84). If you think you may have occupational asthma, visit your doctor as soon as possible.

reactive airways dysfunction syndrome (RADS) Asthma which develops for the first time following a single exposure to high levels of an irritant substance.

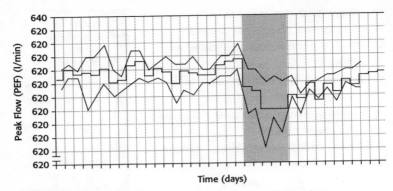

Figure 7.4 Characteristic pattern of lung function in occupational asthma. The daily PEF maximum, minimum and mean are plotted against time. The shaded area represents the five-day period back at work.

my experience

I was always physically fit and played a lot of sport. I was really pleased when I got a job at the aluminium smelter as I enjoyed the physical work, it was well paid and I got lots of time off with shift work. But after a few years I noticed that I started to get breathless at work and coughed and wheezed. It only seemed to occur when I was actually at work or at night after spending a hard day at work. I seemed to be better at the weekend and when I was on holiday. So I went to see my GP who told me that I had developed asthma as a result of my workplace exposure. She started me on treatment, reported my case to Occupational Safety and Health, and said that if I wanted any chance of growing out of the asthma and it not getting worse I had no option but to get another job, which I did. My GP even managed to help get me compensation while I trained for my new job. I was really fortunate as my asthma got better, unlike some of my friends who also developed asthma at the smelter, but stayed on and ended up with really bad asthma.

A useful document is 'Asthma at Work – Your Charter' which sets out ten recommendations to reduce the impact of asthma in the workplace. It provides information on asthma triggers and symptoms, instructions on what to do if someone is having an attack at work and guidance for employers on making the work environment an asthma friendly zone – www.asthma.org.uk/bits/images/Workplace_charter.pdf

Allergic rhinitis

Asthma and **allergic rhinitis** are conditions which often co-exist in the same patient. This is not surprising as the disease process in both conditions is similar, with a person developing asthma if it affects the airways in the lungs and developing rhinitis if it affects the airways in the nose. Allergic rhinitis is often referred to as hay fever, based on the observation that exposure to grass pollens can cause rhinitis. However, this term is seldom used nowadays as grass pollen is only one of many provoking factors in allergic rhinitis and no 'fever' is present. The main symptoms of allergic rhinitis are a blocked and runny nose; **conjunctivitis** may also be present, which causes itchy, runny eyes. Over half of all people with asthma also have rhinitis, which can make asthma worse and add to the impaired quality of life.

Another cause of blocked nasal passages is **nasal polyps** (see Colour Plate 7). Nasal polyps often occur in people with allergic rhinitis and asthma, particularly those who are intolerant of aspirin. Sometimes people with asthma who also have allergic rhinitis and nasal polyps develop a reaction to aspirin which may cause an asthma attack and nasal obstruction.

The treatment of allergic rhinitis usually involves the regular use of drugs that turn off the disease process. Some of the drugs are the same as those

allergic rhinitis
A disorder characterized by inflammation of the nasal passages leading to a blocked and runny nose.

conjunctivitis
An allergic disorder characterized by inflammation of the lining surface of the eyes (conjunctiva), leading to itchy and watering eyes.

nasal polyps
Swelling of nasal tissue that leads to obstruction of the nasal passages.

antihistamine
A medicine which blocks the effects of histamine, which is released by the body as part of an allergic reaction. Antihistamines are widely used to treat rhinitis and conjunctivitis.

used for asthma such as topical inhaled steroids, cromoglycate and leukotriene receptor antagonist drugs; others such as **antihistamines**, which are very effective for allergic rhinitis and conjunctivitis, are comparatively ineffective in treating asthma. In a person with asthma, treatment of co-existing allergic rhinitis is important as it is likely to also lead to an improvement in asthma control.

Sinusitis

sinusitis
A disorder in which there is a bacterial infection of the sinuses.

The major complication of allergic rhinitis is **sinusitis** in which there is recurrent or persisting bacterial infection of the sinuses. The sinuses are the air spaces in the facial bones which connect with the nasal passages. If they are blocked there is a build-up of mucus in the sinuses, which then become infected causing sinusitis (see Colour Plate 6). There are two main forms of sinusitis depending on how long the illness lasts and how frequently it recurs.

Acute sinusitis usually occurs after a cold and presents with fever, facial pain and headaches, nasal congestion and discoloured nasal discharge. The illness normally resolves within a few weeks with a course of antibiotics, nasal decongestants and saline washouts.

Patients with chronic sinusitis suffer from recurrent or persistent symptoms of facial pressure and pain, nasal congestion and discharge, a reduced sense of smell and ear pressure. Most patients with chronic sinusitis suffer from asthma and allergic rhinitis and many also have nasal polyps. Long-term treatment is based on topical nasal steroids to reduce the nasal swelling as well as courses of antibiotics for major infective episodes. Ocassional short courses of oral steriods are sometimes necessory to reduce the nasal and sinus inflammation. Regular nasal washouts with a salt solution can also be helpful. While several commercial saline solutions are available, it is also possible for patients with chronic sinusitis to prepare and administer the solution themselves, as outlined below.

> Saline nasal washouts for sinusitis
>
> ✧ 1 tsp non-iodized sea salt
> ✧ 1 tsp baking soda
>
> Dissolve in one cup of warm water. Put towel around neck. Squirt solution into nose (both sides) from a nasal spray bottle, move head into different positions.

If this approach is not effective, then surgery is the next option. Recently there have been major advances in sinus surgery using an endoscope

my experience

I was getting terrible headaches and a constantly blocked nose. I was referred to an Ear, Nose and Throat surgeon who arranged a CT scan of my sinuses. From this and my symptoms he diagnosed chronic rhinitis and sinusitis. He explained the treatment options, which included steroid nose-drops, antibiotics or surgery. I was surprised to find that with surgery an incision would not be necessary, but instead a fine bendy telescope (called an endoscope) would be inserted up my nose and into my sinuses. The consultant did explain that there were some small risks associated with the procedure, but he said that overall the results were good and recovery rapid. In the end we decided that I should try the nose-drops and reconsider surgery at a later date if they didn't work. So far the steroid nose-drops seem to be keeping my symptoms at bay.

and it is now the surgical treatment of choice in patients who do not respond to standard medical treatment.

Medications to avoid

People with asthma need to be aware that there is a number of medications which can provoke attacks of asthma and therefore should be avoided.

Beta blocker medications

People with asthma should not take **beta blocker medication**, which is commonly prescribed for patients with high blood pressure (hypertension), palpitations, and angina (coronary heart disease). Beta blockers are also prescribed as topical eye solutions for the treatment of glaucoma (a common condition that can cause blindness). The actions of beta blockers are opposite to those of beta agonists, which are used in the treatment of asthma. In contrast to beta agonists, which stimulate the beta receptors and cause airway muscle relaxation, beta blockers cause the airway muscles to constrict, and as a result can provoke an asthma attack in an asthma sufferer. There is a real risk of provoking a life-threatening attack of asthma with beta blockers so they should not be taken by people with asthma. Fortunately there are other drugs that patients with asthma can use in the treatment of hypertension, coronary heart disease and glaucoma.

beta blocker medication

Beta blockers are a group of drugs which are used in the treatment of hypertension, coronary heart disease and glaucoma. They are the opposite of beta agonists.

myth

Beta blocker eye drops are safe in people with asthma as only a small amount is delivered to the eyes and not to the rest of the body.

fact

Beta blocker eye drops have been responsible for the deaths of people with asthma and as a result should not be prescribed to people with asthma.

Non-steroidal anti-inflammatory drugs (NSAIDs)

The **NSAIDs** are a class of drugs (of which aspirin is one) that is used in the treatment of a wide range of illnesses including arthritis, relief of pain and fever and, in the case of aspirin, coronary heart disease. NSAIDs provoke asthma in about one in ten adults with asthma. Although the resulting asthma attack is normally mild, it can occasionally be life-threatening and, consequently, asthmatics should only take NSAIDs with caution. It is worthwhile for a person with asthma to note when they first start taking aspirin or any other NSAIDs, whether it provokes their asthma and, as a result, whether it can be used again with confidence. This is particularly important for patients who also have chronic sinusitis and rhinitis with nasal polyps as they are at greatest risk. Patients with NSAID intolerance often report a combination of asthma, nasal blockage and flushing when they inadvertently take these drugs. Alternative medications such as paracetamol should be used for relief of pain or fever instead.

NSAIDs
A group of drugs used in the treatment of pain, headache, fever and musculoskeletal disorders such as arthritis. The most commonly known NSAID is aspirin which is also one of the key drugs used in the treatment of coronary heart disease.

Q I have asthma – what should I take for a headache?

A Paracetamol is safe for patients with asthma. Aspirin containing pain killers can trigger an asthma attack in some people and are best avoided if possible.

Other medications

There are several other medications that can occasionally cause attacks of asthma. These include some antibiotics, preservatives and colourings that are sometimes included in medications, and royal jelly.

Anaphylaxis

Anaphylaxis is a potentially life-threatening condition that can both mimic and complicate severe asthma. People with asthma are more likely to develop anaphylaxis, particularly those who have severe allergic asthma. The most common cause of anaphylaxis in a person with asthma is a food allergy, in particular an allergy to nuts. Anaphylaxis can also be caused by factors which

anaphylaxis
A generalized allergic reaction which is characterized by flushing and swelling of the body, difficulty in breathing and light-headedness. Anaphylaxis can be a life-threatening condition.

Q **What do I do if I experience anaphylaxis again?**

A At the first signs of anaphylaxis, such as swelling of the face or body, chest tightness, or obstruction in the throat, inject yourself with adrenalin (you should have been provided with an adrenalin kit when you experienced your first episode of anaphylaxis) and phone your doctor or the ambulance for emergency help. Remember the adrenalin should be injected deep into the thigh muscle, not just under the skin.

can provoke asthma such as aspirin and exercise, as well as others such as bee-stings or antibiotics.

One of the difficulties is recognizing anaphylaxis if it also provokes an attack of asthma. Clues to the presence of anaphylaxis are flushing and swelling of the body and mucous membranes (lips and tongue), including the face, a feeling of tightness and obstruction in the throat and/or light-headedness, which occur at the same time as the sudden attack of severe asthma. Hives (urticaria), an itchy, bumpy, swollen rash, which looks like nettle rash, frequently occurs in association with anaphylaxis. If a person with asthma has any of these features of anaphylaxis it is really important to work out what the provoking factor was, so that it can be avoided in the future. It is also important for such people to have a Medic Alert bracelet and ready access to an adrenaline kit (for example, auto-injectable adrenaline syringes such as Epipen®) so they can self-inject adrenaline if anaphylaxis occurs again. Antihistamines are also very helpful but these are of slower onset than the self-administered adrenalin injections. More information on anaphylaxis can be obtained from www.allergy.org.au and from the Anaphylaxis Campaign.

myth
I have had a reaction to peanuts in the past but I haven't had a problem with anaphylaxis for some time so I can probably eat peanuts again.

fact
Even a minute amount of peanut can kill a peanut-allergic person due to anaphylaxis. A person with or without asthma who has a previous episode of anaphylaxis due to a specific food, such as peanuts, must learn how to check whether bought food contains even trace amounts of the specific food and avoid them completely.

Asthma in the elderly

There are a number of problems that relate specifically to the diagnosis and management of asthma in the elderly. It may not be diagnosed because the elderly person may simply accept their symptoms as a sign of old age and nothing more, especially the symptom of breathlessness. If an elderly person with asthma does go to their doctor, the symptoms may be confused with emphysema or chronic bronchitis (also known as COPD, see Chapter 3) due to the symptoms of wheeze, breathlessness and cough which are common to these three disorders. Also, in current or ex-smokers it is common to put all respiratory symptoms down to emphysema or chronic bronchitis, even when they may well be due to asthma. An additional problem is that some older patients have problems performing lung function tests such as peak flow measurements, making the diagnosis of asthma more difficult to make. To address these difficulties, the diagnosis of asthma should be considered in any older person who has episodic breathlessness and wheezing, particularly if they have had wheezing illnesses at some time earlier in their lives.

The management of asthma is the same for the elderly as for younger adults. One issue which is particularly important in the elderly is the choice of drug delivery device, as it must be used correctly. It is always worthwhile for an elderly person with asthma to have their inhaler technique checked regularly by their pharmacist, nurse or doctor. If technique is a problem, there is always the option to use an alternative device, which can be used with ease.

myth
Asthma is not a problem in the elderly.

fact
Asthma is a particular problem in the elderly due to difficulties in its diagnosis and management. It is unfortunate that as a result of these difficulties the death rate for asthma in the elderly is higher than in any other age group (see Figure 7.5).

fact

The flu vaccine is safe for people with asthma. Research has shown that neither an immediate allergic reaction to the vaccine nor a subsequent attack of asthma is likely to occur. This is reassuring as a bout of influenza is an important cause of severe attacks in people with asthma. As a result, the yearly flu vaccine is recommended for people with asthma.

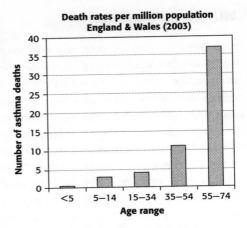

Death rates per million population England & Wales (2003)

Figure 7.5 The death rate from asthma increases dramatically with age.

Another difficulty for the elderly person with asthma is the handling of a severe attack. There is a tendency for elderly patients to delay seeking medical help, as they may not be able to recognize how severe their asthma is, and may not want to bother their doctor. It is therefore crucial that all older people with asthma have a written management plan with instructions on how to recognize a severe attack and what steps to take. As outlined on pages 88–9, medications often prescribed for the elderly, such as beta blockers and NSAIDs, may aggravate asthma.

Vaccinations are another issue in the management of elderly people with asthma. It is important that the elderly asthma sufferer receives a yearly flu vaccine which is likely to reduce the severity of the influenza illness, as well as the risk of hospitalization and death. There is another vaccine called Pneumovax® which protects against pneumonia and is recommended for older people with asthma, and this only needs to be given every five to ten years.

Stopping smoking

People with asthma should not smoke. Research has shown that about one in every two smokers dies prematurely from their smoking and that on average, smokers die about 15 years earlier than non-smokers. The risks are even higher in people with asthma as smoking leads to more frequent severe attacks and loss of effectiveness of inhaled steroids. Furthermore, if a person with asthma also develops emphysema and chronic bronchitis due to smoking, they will be more limited by breathlessness.

The following points may be helpful in motivating people to quit smoking:

- ⬥ It is beneficial to stop smoking at any age, young or old
- ⬥ The earlier smoking is stopped the greater the health gain
- ⬥ Smoking cessation has major and immediate health benefits for smokers of all ages, such as reducing the risk of a heart attack, stroke or lung cancer (to name just a few)
- ⬥ Within one day of quitting the chance of a heart attack decreases
- ⬥ The excess risk of heart disease is reduced by half after one year's abstinence from smoking
- ⬥ After ten years' abstinence the risk of dying almost returns to that of people who never smoked.

Tobacco dependence is a chronic condition that often requires repeated intervention and medical management and support. As part of this process, doctors and other health professionals are trained to provide a quit plan and support to enable the smoker to stop – so ask for their help. The quit plan often involves setting a quit date, anticipating challenges to quitting and removing all tobacco products from the environment around you. Nicotine replacement therapy or a smoking cessation medication called bupropion (Zyban®) are useful treatments that improve the chances of successfully quitting long term.

Most people find it difficult to give up smoking. You can get help by telephoning Ash Quitline:

0800 00 22 00 (England)

0800 84 84 84 (Scotland and Northern Ireland)

0800 169 0169 (Wales).

Advice, support and information about giving up smoking can also be obtained from a number of other sources. Your doctor or nurse should also be able to refer you to a local smoking cessation adivsor or group.

CHAPTER

8

The health care system

Delivery of care

People with asthma deserve regular review as this will result in a better outcome, such as reduced time off school or work and fewer asthma attacks. The improved outcomes can be achieved with regular review from a range of health care professionals in different situations. It is evident that what is actually done would appear to be more important than by whom or where. The type of service available will depend on the particular health care system including the resources and availability of trained staff.

In the United Kingdom over 95 per cent of patients with asthma are cared for by general practitioners and asthma nurses. Asthma clinics that are run by practice nurses with a Diploma in Asthma Care, working with the GP, have been pioneered in the United Kingdom. The nurse-run asthma clinics are run in partnership with the

my experience

I used to see my doctor for my asthma but he always seemed too busy and I never really learnt what to do. I then saw the new asthma nurse at the practice and it was really helpful as she spent a lot of time with me going through what I needed to know and how to monitor and manage my asthma.

Q How do I prioritize the different advice I receive from my doctor?

A The two most important recommendations to follow are:

(1) to make sure you use your preventer therapy regularly to ensure that your asthma is kept under control *(2)* to follow an action plan if your asthma becomes unstable to ensure that any severe attack is properly treated.
To this we can add correct inhaler technique and avoidance of known provoking factors.

GP and have been shown to increase patient satisfaction and reduce the number of severe attacks. It is likely that these improvements are due to the greater amount of time the nurse spends with the patient. There are agreed guidelines to enable doctors and nurses to deliver a consistently high standard of care to their patients.

Clinical review

There is a move towards developing systems where people are offered reviews at a time when they are well, rather than just during a severe attack. Use the following checklist to understand what you need to know about your asthma when you have a clinical review.

Checklist of what patients 'need' to know about their asthma

◇ The diagnosis and how it was made
◇ How to use an inhaler
◇ The difference between relievers and preventers
◇ The importance of regular preventive therapy
◇ Their personal drug regimen
◇ How to use a peak flow meter
◇ How to recognize worsening asthma and what to do
◇ The provoking factors and how to avoid them
◇ When and where they will be followed up.

To assist patients to make the most of their asthma review, Asthma UK has developed an information brochure (see Further help, Chapter 9 for contact details). It is worthwhile reading this document carefully and using it as a reference after the asthma review to remind you of the important issues that were discussed.

In the situation of a severe attack, asthma patients need to know how to recognize when they should obtain medical assistance. Instructions based on both symptoms and/or peak flow recordings should be provided to patients, preferably in written form (see Chapter 6).

Specialist referral

Asthma is a common condition which most family doctors become expert at managing. However, there are several situations when it may be helpful to have a specialist review. If a person with asthma is faced with one of the following situations it would be reasonable to ask for a specialist referral:

Child

◇ Failure to grow properly
◇ Failure to respond to standard treatments
◇ Doubt about the diagnosis.

Adult

◇ Suspected occupational asthma
◇ Oral steroid-dependent asthma
◇ Repeated hospital admissions for asthma
◇ Pregnancy.

CHAPTER

9

Further help

In many countries additional support and information for people with asthma and their carers can be obtained through local or national asthma organizations. These organizations give advice about asthma and its management and provide educational material and resources.

Asthma UK

Asthma UK (formerly the National Asthma Campaign) is an excellent source of independent, professional advice and information to help people increase their understanding of asthma and reduce the effect it has on their lives. Asthma UK has published a series of self-management materials, booklets and printed resources. These materials provide information on a wide range of topics relevant to people with asthma in the UK. Some of these resources include:

Booklets

- ✧ Take control of your asthma
- ✧ Asthma in the under-fives
- ✧ Asthma and me
- ✧ Asthma and my child

Other Resources

- ✧ Asthma Attack Cards
- ✧ Medicine Cards
- ✧ Personal Asthma Action Plans
- ✧ Schools Pack

Factfiles

Factfiles can be found on the Asthma UK website. They cover topics such as:

- ✧ Triggers – asthma and altitude, exercise and asthma, food reactions and asthma, housing location and asthma, indoor environment and asthma, low allergen gardens
- ✧ Symptoms and treatments – nebulizers, non-drug approaches to managing your asthma, prescription charges, severe asthma symptoms and how to control them, vaccination and immunization
- ✧ Children and young people – diet and asthma in babies, severe asthma at school, youth groups
- ✧ Finances and financial assistance – financial assistance, solving housing problems
- ✧ Statistics and research – Asthma Audit 2001: out in the open, searching for new information about asthma.

Asthma Charter

Asthma UK also works with the NHS, health care professionals and government to raise awareness about the seriousness of asthma and the necessary standards of care. This has led to the drafting and implementation of the Asthma Charter (see Figure 9.1) which outlines the treatment that people with this condition have a right to expect.

Booklets and other printed resources can be ordered by UK residents from:

Asthma UK
Summit House, 70 Wilson Street,
London, EC2A 2DB
Telephone: 020 7786 5000
Email: info@asthma.org.uk

For factfiles and further information visit Asthma UK's website: www.asthma.org.uk

UK residents can also call or email an asthma nurse for independent, specialist advice:
Telephone: 08457 01 02 03
Email: asthma.org.uk/adviceline

The Asthma Charter

The Asthma Charter is a **charter for change**.

It describes the quality of care you, as a person with asthma, should receive from your National Health Service. It aims to ensure that everyone who works in the NHS and government gives asthma the priority it deserves.

*As a person with asthma **I have a right to:***

1 High-quality treatment, care and information from asthma-trained health care professionals who know about best practice and the latest evidence.

2 Access to a doctor or nurse who has had specific asthma training, at either my own GP practice or in my local area.

3 Have my asthma quickly and accurately diagnosed, with referral to a respiratory specialist if necessary.

4 A full and open discussion with my doctor or nurse about the best asthma treatments for me, including side effects, regardless of the cost of treatment.

5 Be shown how to use the devices needed to keep my asthma under control (e.g. inhalers and spacers).

6 Discuss and agree my own asthma action plan with my doctor or nurse so that I can keep my asthma under control.

7 Have my asthma reviewed about once a year (more frequently if I have severe asthma symptoms), at a time convenient to me, or in the case of my children, every six months.

8 Be referred to a respiratory specialist if my asthma is becoming unmanageable and to be admitted to a specialist respiratory unit if I need to go to hospital.

9 Have follow-up appointments made with my doctor and my specialist before I am discharged from hospital or leave A&E.

10 Expect any people working in the NHS that I need to contact to be aware of the serious risks I face if my asthma symptoms are deteriorating (e.g. practice receptionists, ambulance personnel and NHS Direct staff).

Figure 9.1 The Asthma Charter.

Other sources

There are numerous other asthma organizations which provide advice and information, both nationally and internationally. Sources of further educational material, including links to several asthma websites, can be found at www.ginasthma.com. A gateway to all the asthma and allergy information on the web can be found on www.allallergy.net

Below is list of some of the useful websites that are available.

Allergy and Allergies Agency
www.allergy-network.co.uk

Allergy and Asthma Network/Mothers of Asthmatics Inc.
www.aanma.org

Allergy Asthma and Immunology Online (US)
www.allergy.mcg.edu

American Academy of Allergy, Asthma and Immunology
www.aaaai.org

Anaphylaxis Campaign
www.anaphylaxis.org.uk

Asthma and Respiratory Foundation of New Zealand
www.asthmanz.co.nz

Asthma Australia
www.asthmaaustralia.org.au

Asthma Learning Lab
www.asthmalearninglab.com

Asthma Society of Canada
www.asthma.ca

Asthma UK
www.asthma.org.uk

AsthmaWeb
www.asthmaweb.net

British Lung Foundation
www.lunguk.org/index.htm

British Thoracic Society
www.brit-thoracic.org.uk

Canadian Lung Association
www.lung.ca/asthma

Canadian Network for Asthma Care (Canada)
www.cnac.net

European Federation of Asthma and Allergy Associations
www.efanet.org

Health and Safety Executive's Asthma website
www.hse.gov.uk/asthma

National Asthma Council (Australia)
www.nationalasthma.org.au

National Heart, Lung and Blood Institute (US)
www.nhlbi.nih.gov

Occupational Asthma
www.hse.gov.uk/asthma/genguide.htm

World Health Organization
www.who.int

The following books on asthma can also be recommended:

Asthma at Your Fingertips, second edition, Levy M, Hilton S and Barnes G. Class Publishing, London 1997.

Asthma: Ask the Experts, National Asthma Training Centre. Class Publishing, London 1997.

Manual of Asthma Management, second edition, O'Byrne P and Thomson NC (eds). W B Saunders Company Ltd, London 2001.

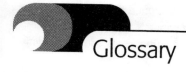

Glossary

airway lumen
The space within the tubes through which air flows into and out of the lungs.

airways
The tubes that carry air in and out of the lungs.

allergen
A substance that may provoke an allergic response in a susceptible person. Common allergens include house-dust mites, grass pollen and cat dander.

allergic rhinitis
A disorder characterized by inflammation of the nasal passages leading to a blocked and runny nose.

anaphylaxis
A generalized allergic reaction which is characterized by flushing and swelling of the body, difficulty in breathing and light-headedness. Anaphylaxis can be a life-threatening condition.

antihistamine
A medicine which blocks the effects of histamine, which is released by the body as part of an allergic reaction. Antihistamines are widely used to treat rhinitis and conjunctivitis.

asthma action plan
A written plan that provides patients with guidelines for the assessment and management of asthma.

asthma attack
An episode of severe asthma in which a person has difficulty breathing. The cause of the attack and its presentation may vary.

beta blocker
Beta blockers are a group of drugs which are used in the treatment of hypertension, coronary heart disease and glaucoma. They are the opposite of beta agonists.

bronchospasm
The contraction of the airway (bronchial) muscles that leads to a narrowing of the airway lumen in asthma.

bronchodilator
A medication used to treat asthma symptoms, also known as a reliever. Bronchodilators work by relaxing the muscles around the airways and making breathing easier.

bronchodilator therapy
Medications that relax the airway muscle, leading to relief of airflow obstruction and symptoms of asthma over short periods. Bronchodilator therapy is often called 'reliever' therapy because it is used to relieve asthma symptoms.

bronchial hyper-responsiveness
The enhanced sensitivity of the airways in asthma, causing bronchospasm in response to irritants that do not normally affect people without asthma.

chlorofluorocarbons (CFCs)
The propellants used in metered dose inhalers which are damaging to the ozone layer.

chronic bronchitis
A disease which is characterized by the over-production of phlegm in response to long-term exposure to irritants (such as smoking). People with chronic bronchitis have a persistent cough with phlegm, as well as wheezing.

chronic obstructive pulmonary disease (COPD)
A group of slowly progressive respiratory conditions resulting from long-term exposure to irritants to the lung such as smoking. COPD is characterized by airflow obstruction that does not fully reverse and is associated with infective episodes, especially in the winter months.

compliance

The extent to which a person's behaviour, in terms of taking medication or making lifestyle changes, coincides with the advice from a doctor. It assumes that a correct diagnosis has been made, that the doctor's advice is appropriate and that the patient is able to follow the advice.

concordance

The extent to which an agreed plan is followed by the patient. In contrast to compliance, concordance shows respect for the aims of both the doctor and the patient and means that there has been a negotiated agreement between the two.

conjunctivitis

A disorder characterized by inflammation of the lining surface of the eyes (conjunctiva), leading to itchy and watering eyes.

dry powder inhaler

A device that automatically releases a medication as a dry powder when a patient breathes in through the mouthpiece. Such devices are also referred to as 'breath actuated inhalers'.

eczema

A skin condition that makes the skin dry and itchy.

emphysema

A disease in which the lung is progressively destroyed due to exposure to irritants (such as smoking). It is characterized by breathlessness which limits daily activities.

FEV_1

The forced expiratory volume in one second – the amount of air that can be forced out of the lungs in one second.

guided self-management

Management approach in which patients control their own condition with guidance from the health care professional.

house-dust mite

Tiny creatures that live in the dust that builds up around the house, in particular in mattresses, carpets and soft furnishings. Most people with asthma are allergic to the faeces from the house-dust mite.

hydrofluorocarbons (HFAs)
The propellants that have replaced CFCs in metered dose inhalers (MDIs) due to their lack of harmful effects on the ozone layer.

immunoglobulin E (IgE)
The antibody which is involved in allergic responses.

inflammation
The process whereby the body responds to injury or irritation. It involves a complex series of events. Inflammation is the underlying problem in asthma. It is the main reason the airways in asthma are 'twitchy', responding to triggers that irritate them.

inhaler
A device that delivers asthma medication to the airways. There are several different types of inhalers including the metered dose inhaler and dry powder inhaler.

metered dose inhaler (MDI)
An MDI is the usual device which people with asthma use to deliver their medications. When the canister is pressed it releases the medication as an aerosol, which the patient breathes into their lungs, where it exerts its effect.

nasal polyps
Swelling of the nasal tissue that leads to obstruction of the nasal passages.

nebulizer
A nebulizer is a device which pumps air through a liquid (in a pot), thereby creating a fine mist of aerosol droplets. If the solution is an asthma medication, the resulting mist can be breathed in by a patient with asthma through a face mask or mouthpiece.

nocturnal asthma
Asthma symptoms which occur at night. It is a sign that asthma is not under adequate control, even if asthma symptoms are not a problem during the day.

NSAIDs
A group of drugs used in the treatment of pain, headache, fever and musculoskeletal disorders such as arthritis. The most commonly known NSAID is aspirin which is also one of the key drugs used in the treatment of coronary heart disease.

occupational asthma	Asthma that develops as a direct result of repeated exposure to substances in the workplace such as fumes or dusts.
osteoporosis	A condition characterized by thin bones which can result in fractures. Osteoporosis can be caused by long-term oral steroid therapy and is treated by a class of medications called bisphosphonates.
peak flow	The maximum speed at which air can be forced out of the lungs. It is a sensitive measure of the severity of the obstruction to the flow of air in a person with asthma.
peak flow meter	A device which measures the maximum speed at which air can be forced out of the lungs.
pollen	The tiny grains given off by grasses, flowers and trees. Most people with rhinitis, and many with asthma, are allergic to pollens.
pre-menstrual asthma	A cyclical worsening of asthma control in the week prior to the menstrual period.
prevalence	The proportion of people with a condition in a defined population.
preventive drug	A medication which reduces the severity of asthma when taken regularly over a prolonged period. Preventive drugs work by turning off the underlying disease process in asthma.
preventive therapy	Treatment that turns off the disease process in asthma, leading to improvements in asthma control with long-term use.
primary prevention	Intervention made before any evidence of disease to prevent the disease from developing.
reactive airways dysfunction syndrome (RADS)	Asthma which develops for the first time following a single exposure to high levels of an irritant substance.
reversible airflow obstruction	Airflow obstruction that comes and goes over short periods, being worse with provoking stimuli (such as cold air) and resolving with treatment (such as inhaled bronchodilator).

rhinitis	An allergic condition of the nasal passages that causes a blocked and/or runny nose and sneezing.
secondary prevention	Intervention made after the onset of disease to reduce its impact.
sinusitis	A disorder in which there is a bacterial infection of the sinuses.
skin prick test	A test to find out whether a person is sensitive to specific allergens. Drops of allergen are placed on the skin, the skin is then pricked through the allergen solution, and the size of the resulting skin swelling is measured.
spacer	A spacer is a chamber which holds the medication for the person to breathe in. An MDI is inserted in one end of the spacer; the medication is released as an aerosol from the MDI into the spacer; the patient with asthma breathes in the aerosol through a one-way valve at the other end of the spacer.
sputum	The thick mucus which is coughed up by a person. It is also commonly called phlegm.
steroids	A group of chemicals that is produced naturally in the body by the adrenal gland. There are many types of steroids that are used for medical purposes. In asthma steroids are used to reduce the underlying disease process, the inflammation of the airways.
symptom	A sensation experienced by an individual as a result of an illness or problem. The symptoms of asthma include breathlessness, wheezing, coughing and chest tightness.
viral respiratory tract infection	An infection of the respiratory tract caused by a virus. The site and severity of the illness may vary depending on the specific virus, ranging from a runny nose due to the common cold virus to an illness with fever, aching, breathlessness and coughing due to the influenza virus.

wheeze

A whistling sound made by a patient who has airflow obstruction when breathing. In a person with asthma wheezing is high-pitched, and is usually heard when breathing out, although if airflow obstruction is severe it may also occur when breathing in. If a person with very severe asthma stops wheezing, this is a serious sign as it means the airways have narrowed so much that there is not enough air passing through them to make the wheezing sound.

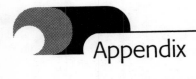

Appendix

Peak flow diary

Use your peak flow meter first thing in the morning and in the evening before your treatment.

Take a peak flow reading by putting the marker to zero, taking a deep breath, sealing your lips around the mouthpiece, and then blowing as hard and as fast as you can into the device.

Make a note of the reading. Repeat this process three times. Mark the best of the three readings with a cross on the peak flow chart opposite.

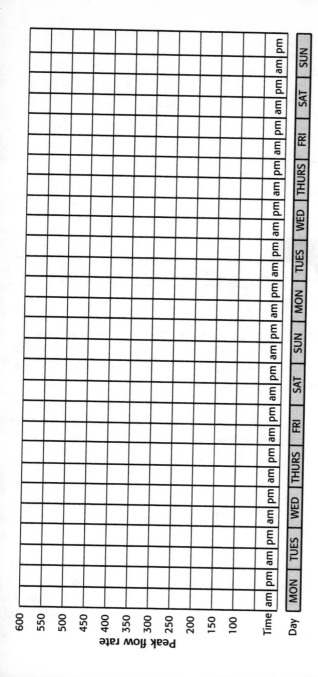

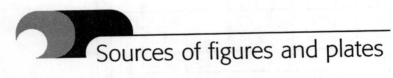

Sources of figures and plates

Figure 1.1
World map of the prevalence of clinical asthma. From Masoli M, Fabian D, Holt S and Beasley R, Global Burden of Asthma Report. Global Initiative for Asthma (GINA), US National Heart, Lung and Blood Institute, National Institutes of Health and the World Health Organization, 2004; p.122.

Figure 1.2
The reduction in the death rate from asthma in the United Kingdom since 1990. Derived from National Statistics UK. www.statistics.gov.uk/downloads/theme_health/Dh2_30/DH2No30.pdf

Figure 1.3
The allergic march. From 'Eczema and contact dermatitis – pathophysiology', in *Allergy*, Holgate S T and Church M K (eds). Gower Medical Publishing, London 1993; p.23.8 (Fig. 23.16).

Figure 2.1
Airways in the normal state (left) and in asthma (right), demonstrating the narrowing of the airway lumen due to thickening of the airway wall and mucus, which leads to a greater resistance to the flow of air in and out of the lungs. From Jeffery P K, 'Pathology of asthma', in *Respiratory Medicine*,

third edition, volume 2, Gibson G J, Geddes D M, Costabel U, Sterk P J and Corrin B (eds). Elsevier Science Limited, 2003; p.1266 (Fig. 48.3.1).

Figure 2.2

The hyperresponsive airways in asthma respond to a wide range of provoking factors. From 'Asthma – pathophysiology', in *Allergy*, Holgate S T and Church M K (eds). Gower Medical Publishing, London 1993; p.13.3 (Fig. 13.5).

Figure 2.3

A house-dust mite magnified 500 times. From *Allergy*, Holgate S T and Church M K (eds). Gower Medical Publishing, London 1993; p.1.4 (Fig. 1.6).

Figure 2.4

Proportions of asthmatic children sensitized to the common allergens. From Djukanović R and Holgate S T, *An Atlas of Asthma*. Parthenon Publishing Group, London 1999; p.61 (Fig. 65).

Figure 3.1

The peak flow record of an untreated patient with asthma shows characteristic variability, being worse in the early morning and better in the late afternoon. From Masoli M and Beasley R, *Diagnosis and Management of Adult Asthma*. The Medicine Publishing Company Ltd 2003; p.63 (Fig. 2). Originally from Clark T J H (ed.), *Bronchodilator Therapy: The Basis of Asthma and Chronic Obstructive Airways Disease Management*. ADIS Press, Auckland 1994.

Figure 4.1

A peak flow meter. Courtesy of Lesley Baillie.

Figure 4.2

A spirometer. Garo/Phanie/Rex Features.

Figure 4.3

Standard tables for peak flow in children (top). From Godfrey S *et al.*, Br J Dis Chest; 1970; vol. 64: pp.15–24 and adults (bottom). A total of 95 per cent of all children will have a peak flow value between 2SD and −2SD lines. From Gregg I, Nunn A J. BMJ 1989; vol. 298: pp.168–70. *Guidelines on the Management of Asthma*, THORAX, The Journal of the British Thoracic Society, March 1993; 48; 2: 520–1.

Figure 5.1
A nebulizer. Courtesy of Lesley Baillie.

Figure 5.2
Stepwise management, in which patients step up or step down depending on asthma control.

Figure 5.3
A metered dose inhaler (MDI). Courtesy of Lesley Baillie.

Figure 5.4
An Accuhaler. Courtesy of Lesley Baillie.

Figure 5.5
MDI with spacer.

Figure 6.1
Use of a self-management plan in a patient with deteriorating asthma. From Masoli M and Beasley R, *Diagnosis and Management of Adult Asthma*. The Medicine Publishing Company Ltd 2003.

Figure 6.2
The New Zealand Asthma and Respiratory Foundation asthma action plan. From the *New Zealand Asthma and Respiratory Foundation*, www.asthmanz.co.nz.

Figure 7.1
A mother giving her young child asthma medication from an MDI and spacer. From *Asthma at your Fingertips*, p.72 (Fig. 2.10).

Figure 7.2
An MDI can be used through a plastic cup as an alternative to a spacer. From *Asthma at your Fingertips*, p.78 (Fig. 2.12).

Figure 7.3
A person with asthma usually experiences an improvement in their lung function (FEV_1 or PEF) when they begin exercising. However, if the person stops exercising after about five minutes, their lung function gets worse as they experience a worsening in their asthma. This is called exercise-induced asthma. From Djukanović R and Holgate S T, *An Atlas of Asthma*. Parthenon Publishing Group, London 1999; p.63 (Fig. 69).

Figure 7.4

Characteristic pattern of lung function in occupational asthma: the shaded area represents the five-day period back at work. From Djukanović R and Holgate S T, *An Atlas of Asthma*. Parthenon Publishing Group, London 1999; p.73 (Fig. 82).

Figure 7.5

The death rate from asthma increases dramatically with age. Derived from National Statistics UK. www.statistics.gov.uk/downloads/theme_health/ Dh2_30/DH2No30.pdf.

Figure 9.1

The Asthma Charter. Provided by Asthma UK, 2005.

Colour Plate 1

Eczema on the back of a child's legs. From 'Eczema and contact dermatitis – diagnosis and treatment', in *Allergy*, Holgate S T and Church M K (eds). Gower Medical Publishing, London 1993; p.24.6 (Fig. 24.12).

Colour Plate 2

Mucus casts from airways coughed up by a person with asthma. From Clark T and Rees J (eds), *Practical Management of Asthma*. Martin Dunitz Ltd, London 1985; p.18.

Colour Plate 3

Section of a lung from a patient who died from asthma, showing the occlusion of airways by mucus (arrows). From Djukanović R and Holgate S T, *An Atlas of Asthma*. Parthenon Publishing Group, London 1999; p.28 (Fig. 18).

Colour Plate 4

The airways of (left) a healthy person and (right) a person with asthma. The redness and swelling of the airways in asthma is evident. From 'Asthma – pathophysiology', in *Allergy*, Holgate S T and Church M K (eds). Gower Medical Publishing, London 1993; p.13.1 (Fig. 13.24).

Colour Plate 5

Skin prick tests for common allergies. Strong responses to house dust mite (DP), grass pollen (P), cat dander (C) and positive control (H) are present. From Djukanović R and Holgate S T, *An Atlas of Asthma*. Parthenon Publishing Group, London 1999; p.75 (Fig. 84).

Colour Plate 6

CT scan of sinusitis in which the infected mucus is evident, filling the right nasal cavity (arrow). From P O'Byrne, N C Thomson (eds), *Manual of Asthma Management*, W B Saunders Company Ltd, London; p.698 (Figure 39.6(b)).

Colour Plate 7

A normal nasal passage (left) and a nasal polyp blocking the nasal passage in a person with asthma (right). From 'Allergic rhinitis – diagnosis and treatment,' in *Allergy*, Holgate S T and Church M K (eds). Gower Medical Publishing, London 1993; p.18.2 (Figs 18.1 and 18.2).

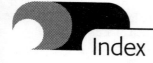

Index

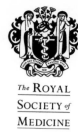

The ROYAL
SOCIETY *of*
MEDICINE

The Royal Society of Medicine (RSM) is an independent medical charity with a primary aim to provide continuing professional development for qualified medical and health-related professionals. The public benefits from health care professionals who have received high quality and relevant education from the RSM.

The Society celebrated its bicentenary in 2005. Each year it arranges and holds over 400 meetings for health care professionals across a wide range of medical subjects. In order to aid education and further training the Society also has the largest postgraduate medical library in Europe – based in central London together with online access to specialist databases. The RSM Press, the Society's publishing arm, publishes books and journals principally aimed at the medical profession.

A number of conferences and events are held each year for the public as well as members of the Society. These include the successful 'Medicine and me' series, designed to bring together patients, their carers and the medical profession. The RSM's Open and History of Medicine Sections also arrange meetings on a regular basis which can be attended by the public.

In addition to the lectures and training provided by the RSM, members of the Society also have access to club facilities including accommodation and a restaurant. The conference and meeting facilities of the RSM were refurbished for their bicentenary and are available to the public for hire for meetings and seminars. Chandos House, a beautifully restored Georgian townhouse, designed by Robert Adam, is also now available to hire for training, receptions and weddings (as it has a civil wedding licence).

To find out more about the Royal Society of Medicine and the work it undertakes please visit www.rsm.ac.uk or call 020 7290 2991. For more information about RSM Press, please visit www.rsmpress.co.uk.